The Unsuspecting Connection between Binge Eating Disorder and Body Dysmorphic Disorder and how you can stop it dead in its track

By Ted Dawson

Table of Contents

Introduction

You or your loved one may have Binge Eating Disorder and/or Body Dysmorphic Disorder and that is why you may be reading this helpful book. Did you know that these conditions are related? Yes they are and they not only affect your quality of life, but your well-being as well. Fortunately, they are both curable. In this book you will find the solutions to these problems because it has all the resources you need. It shows you the steps to take, to ensure your recovery.

Binge Eating Disorder is related to Body Dysmorphic Disorder although most people may not know this. That is why tackling the two conditions together is the only way to stop them from plaguing your life. This book gives you important tips of how you can overcome these conditions and live a happy and meaningful life. You can stop any of these conditions right away starting today, if you follow what we have recommended.

This book reveals to you, the steps which you can take to overcome Binge Eating Disorder and Body Dysmorphic Disorder as well as other conditions associated with these problems. As you overcome these conditions you will discover that, other problems start to disappear. Do you want to live a healthy life free from compulsive and obsessive habits? Read this book and you will overcome these disorders and live a happy and vibrant life.

Chapter 1:
What is Body Dysmorphic Disorder?

Many questions arise about Body Dysmorphic Disorder (BDD). What is Body Dysmorphic Disorder? What are the symptoms? How is it diagnosed? What causes it? How can it be cured? You will find the answers to all these questions and many others, in this chapter and the following chapters. You may be suffering from BDD and you don't know much about it. You may have symptoms that you find difficult to ignore. Maybe that is what led you to this book, or you want to help a loved one, find solutions to the problem. You may also read this book to help you prevent this condition. Whatever your intentions are, you are at the right place at the right time. Learning about this disorder will pave the way to recovery. You will find solutions to your problems as you read on.

What is BDD?

Body Dysmorphic Disorder (BDD) is also known as body dysmorphia or dysmorphic syndrome. What is it? It's a mental disorder that affects a person's body image although it portrays itself as a medical illness. Another term for it is dysmorphophobia which is the fear of having a deformity. It is the belief that, the person's own appearance is defective or has a flaw, which should be hidden or fixed. Sufferers have a distorted self-image about their body. They fret over their physical appearance more than usual, and they often hide from other people to keep the disorder a secret. If you or your loved one thinks you have BDD, you should not suffer in secret. You should know that, there is a solution to this problem and you can be cured. That is why you shouldn't hide it. Get help immediately and overcome it. As you read this book, you will gain confidence to beat it in its own track and we will show you how to do it, if you read on.

BDD is a distinct mental disorder whereby a person has symptoms of a medical illness, but the symptoms cannot be fully explained by an actual physical disorder. That is why it can take long to be rectified if you don't reveal it. The disorder affects a person's body image as we shall see and that is why it is related to eating disorders especially binge eating disorder. People with BDD are preoccupied with an actual or imagined physical defect that others most often cannot see. '

Most of us have something which we may not like about our appearance. It may be the eyes, nose, chin, teeth, breasts, hips or anything else. That is why you are not alone in this, and there is nothing to be ashamed of. We may have too small or too big eyes, a crooked nose, big ears or a rough spotty face with acne. Usually, we fret about it and move on with our lives. We don't get obsessed with the appearance because it's normal. That means that, it doesn't interfere with our daily lives or our well-being although at one time or another we may worry about it. But people who have Body Dysmorphic Disorder (BDD) spend a lot of time thinking about their flaws whether they are real or perceived. They spend hours each day, looking at the mirror or avoiding it. They regularly worry about how they look and how others perceive them.

These people are unable to control their negative thoughts and as much as they may seek reassurance and get it, oftentimes they don't believe those who reassure them that they look just fine. Are you one of those people? Don't worry. Look around you and see people who are just like you or even worse, but they are just happy and content. The way you look doesn't define you. You are more than that. You may even be admired by many people who wish they were you. If you think you have flaws which you may not have, start by appreciating yourself. Even if you have them, they may be minor and unnoticeable and it doesn't help you much, if you keep worrying about them. These are not physical problems about your problems but distorted beliefs about your body image. Yes, that is what they are. These negative thoughts, feelings and behavior may have caused you emotional distress and interfered with your daily life. Stop them right away and we will show you how.

When people suffer from BDD, they get preoccupied with the flaw or defect and they constantly look at themselves in the mirror for a long time or avoid it altogether. Does this sound familiar to you? They obsess over their appearance and body image so often, in fact, for many hours in a day at times over 2 hours. This obsession with their body image causes distress, and this impacts their ability to function well in their daily life. Their normal functioning suffers and that is why it is a disorder. They may miss going to work or to school, avoid social situations and they isolate themselves, even from their family and friends, because they become fearful that others will notice their flaws.

As a result, these people view themselves as ugly or they feel their appearance is shameful. They may be pretty and attractive but they will not see it or believe those who tell them the truth. They may avoid social exposure and social interactions with other people. They may feel they don't want to be seen even by family members and close friends. These people may try to improve their appearance by turning to cosmetic surgery. Some undergo unnecessary plastic surgeries to correct their perceived imperfections although they may never find satisfaction with the results because the problem is not physical but mental. They may exercise excessively to try to fix their appearance but they are never satisfied.

BDD shares some features with Binge Eating Disorder and other eating disorders as well as obsessive compulsive disorder. The similarity is the concern people with these disorders have about their body image. However, a person with a type of eating disorder is more concerned about weight and shape. This is the shape of the entire body while a person who has BDD is concerned about a specific body part like the nose, thighs, breasts or buttocks.

This condition becomes severe if it is not treated, and it can be so severe that, it affects the sufferer's life, well-being, and the ability to function well. Fortunately, in Chapter 2 you will discover the steps you can take to overcome BDD. You will know what you can do, the different types of treatments and important tips about coping or overcoming this disorder.

Prevalence of BDD

BDD is a relatively common mental disorder which affects over 2% of the population although the actual figures may not be known because people hide about it. It is generally thought to affect both men and women equally. This means that, it can occur in anyone whether it is a man or woman. There are therefore no discrepancies about BDD prevalence in relation to gender. Where there are discrepancies, they must have arisen due to research inconsistencies about the diagnosis which were reported before the creation of a standardized questionnaire.

BDD can occur in children as well as in adults. Although the cause of BDD is not known for sure, it is believed to begin during adolescence when a lot of changes take place in the body. The cause may not be fully understood but there are strong indicators that, BDD may have strong links to bullying and abuse as well as other social aspects, at a young age. Such social aspects include the expectation to look attractive as is prevalent in the society today. This may manifest itself as BDD. Genetics may also be a crucial factor when determining those susceptible to this condition.

Studies have shown that:

- 8% of BDD sufferers have a close relative who also has or had the mental disorder.

- 7% of BDD sufferers have a close relative who has or had Obsessive Compulsive Behavior (OCD).

Symptoms of Body Dysmorphic Disorder

It is important to understand the symptoms of BDD whether you are the sufferer or a close relative or friend to the sufferer. This is the only way you will know what you need to change, in order to overcome the problem. The best thing is that, we will walk with you in this process. You will understand yourself and you will follow proven methods that others have followed and become free from this mental disorder.

It is normal to fret about your body appearance, most of us do, but, when does it become an obsession? When do you know that you have taken things too far beyond the normal range?

People who have Body Dysmorphic Disorder suffer from obsessions about their appearance that can last for many hours or even a whole day. They find it hard to resist or to control these obsessions. This makes it difficult for them to be able to focus on anything else such as work or academics, except their own imperfections. This may lead to problems at work or school, low self-esteem, being homebound and avoidance of social situations.

Rituals and Routines

BDD sufferers try to hide or improve their real or imagined flaws by performing compulsive or repetitive rituals and routines although this only gives them temporary relief.

They may be involved in:

- camouflaging with excess makeup, clothing, body position and hair styles

- comparing their body appearance with others

- looking in a mirror for hours

- avoiding mirrors altogether

- changing clothes excessively

- excessive grooming

- skin picking to smooth it

- exercising excessively to lose weight

- seeking cosmetic surgery repeatedly

Signs and Symptoms

The following are the signs and symptoms of body dysmorphic disorder:

- ➢ Being preoccupied with your physical appearance and obsessing about your body features as well as having extreme self-consciousness. You may believe that, others notice your physical appearance in a negative way which may not be true.

- ➢ Frequently examining yourself in the mirror for over 2 hours, or doing the opposite, avoiding the mirror altogether. Excessive grooming may include hair plucking or skin picking to smooth it, or exercising excessively to improve the flaw such as body weight with little or no success.

➤ Having a strong belief that, you have a flaw, an abnormality or a defect in your appearance which you interpret as ugliness or shameful although it may not be. You may have a need to grow a beard or to wear excessive makeup or clothing to cover up the perceived flaws.

➤ You may obsess over any part of your body. The most common areas of concern for people with BDD include:

- Skin – complexion concerns about acne, wrinkles, scars, blemishes and vein appearance.

- Hair – presence of head and body hair, as well as absence of it i.e. thinning and baldness.

- Face - facial features such as the size and shape of the nose, eyes, lips, eyelids, mouth, chin and others.

- Body weight – weight, muscle tone and size, as well as presence or lack of muscles.

- Other concerns include the size of breasts, thighs, buttocks, and the smell of body odor. While many BDD sufferers are preoccupied with their facial features, it is common for other body features like breasts to be viewed as the perceived defect.

➢ You may avoid social situations and feel the need to stay in the house away from the public. You may feel reluctant to appear on photos.

➢ You may have the need to seek reassurance about your physical appearance from others although you may not believe what you are told.

➢ You may seek frequent cosmetic procedures such as plastic surgery with little or no satisfaction with the results.

➢ Comparing your appearance with that of others and feeling discontent with how you look.

➢ In the most severe cases sufferers may have suicidal thoughts and even attempt suicide.

When you have BDD you may be so convinced about your real or perceived flaws that, you imagine your body image as negative. This may not be true but you believe it is true no matter how much someone else tries to convince you that it's not. This concern about the perceived flaw can easily dominate your life to the extent that, you develop extreme self-consciousness.

A person with BDD may be concerned about any part of their body but usually it is the face. People are different. Some people are very precise about a particular feature like the nose or skin while others have a general perception of their ugliness. However, both groups frequently attach strong personal meanings and interpretations or beliefs about their appearance. For example, one person may believe that her crooked nose makes her unlovable while another may think that she generally looks ugly.

These people usually expect others to have the same beliefs about them, but it is only in their mind. When they believe that other people evaluate them negatively, just because of their physical appearance, they feel isolated and they avoid social interactions.

Warning signs of someone with Body Dysmorphic Disorder

There are certain things that can indicate that someone has BDD. Whether you are the one having BDD or someone you know, you can notice these warning signs which should convince you or your loved one to seek help. You can also offer help or convince your loved one to seek treatment. However, anyone can overcome this problem on their own if it is detected early.

- People with BDD engage in repetitive and time-consuming behaviors such as looking in a mirror for too long, picking at their skin, hiding or covering up the real or imagined defect constantly.

- They ask for reassurance from others. This is to reassure them that, the defect is not visible and most times it's not or it's not too obvious as they believe.

- They measure or touch the real or imagined defect several times in a day. This may involve weighing themselves on the scale if they are over-weight, measuring their waistline and hips excessively, to see if they have lost weight.

- They usually experiences problems at work or school, or in their relationships due to the inability to stop focusing about their real or perceived defect.

- They feel too anxious when they are around people and may be too self-conscious which will make them avoid going out in public.

- They may also repeatedly consult with medical experts such as plastic surgeons or dermatologists, to find ways to improve their appearance.

Diagnoses

Diagnoses of Body Dysmorphic Disorder, involves meeting the symptom criteria in the Diagnostic and Statistical Manual of Mental Disorders (DSM) that is contained in the manual, published by the American Psychiatric Association. This is used by mental health providers to diagnose BDD and other mental illnesses.

Diagnostic criteria for Body Dysmorphic Disorder

Body Dysmorphic Disorder is diagnosed when the following 3 criteria are met:

- First Criteria: Preoccupation

- Second Criteria: Distress

- Third Criteria: Not Something Else

1. <u>First Criteria: Preoccupation</u> - First of all, the sufferers must be preoccupied with either a real or imagined flaw or defect in their own appearance. If the defect is real, the sufferers become excessively concerned about the minor physical anomaly.

2. <u>Second Criteria: Distress</u> - Secondly, there should be distress. The sufferers must be distressed to a large extent by their preoccupation or their excessive concern about their appearance. This leads to impairment about their work-related and social activities which they are supposed to participate in.

3. Third Criteria: Not Something Else - Thirdly, the distress should not be due to something else.

How Is BDD Diagnosed?

Diagnosis of BDD is difficult and it is not fully recorded. Many people who have this condition don't report it and they keep it as a secret because of the shame that it causes them. This makes diagnosis of BDD difficult. Most experts and medical practitioners agree that, many of these cases go unrecognized. People who suffer from this disorder oftentimes feel embarrassed about it and about their obsessions. They therefore feel reluctant to reveal their concern and behavior to their doctors.

Since this condition cannot be easily diagnosed like a physical condition, it can go unnoticed for many years. In some people it may never be diagnosed. One of the ways BDD raises a red flag and may be detected by doctors is when the patient seeks plastic surgery repeatedly for the same perceived physical defect and fails to get satisfied with the results.

How the diagnosis is carried out

The doctor will most likely start the evaluation of BDD, by taking the medical history of the patient, including that of the family because the condition can be caused by genetic predisposition. This may be followed by a physical exam. The doctor will focus on certain areas of the body which many BDD patients are concerned about. The doctor will also have an observation of the patient's behavior looking for signs and symptoms. If the doctor suspects that there is likelihood of BDD, he or she may refer the person to a psychologist, a psychiatrist, trained therapist or a specialized health care professional.

There are health care professionals even nurses who are specially trained to diagnose and treat these mental disorders. The professional makes a diagnosis which is based on his or her assessment of the sufferer's behavior, attitudes, and symptoms.

The following tests may be carried out:

Physical exam – helps to identify other symptoms that are associated with BDD symptoms.

Lab tests – may be recommended by your doctor. The lab tests depend on your overall health and the problems you may have which are associated with your symptoms.

Psychological evaluation – the doctor or mental health provider will want to know about your symptoms, thoughts, feelings and behaviors. If you have self-harm thoughts, you should not hide them. Discuss about them so solutions can be found. This is for your own benefit.

About half of the people who are diagnosed with BDD spend over 3 hours in a day or the whole day attempting to hide or correct the real or perceived flaw. If this flaw is perceived then it is not a reality so it is easy to deal with it. If the flaw is real, it is usually minor, although it is oftentimes exaggerated. You should be careful about how you perceive yourself because the distress caused by BDD can affect your quality of life. It can impair your work, social and academic functioning, and lead to social isolation.

Under-diagnosis of BDD

Body Dysmorphic Disorder is usually under-diagnosed although it has been present and it has been described for many years all over the world. The knowledge of BDD is still not widespread among general practitioners and clinicians. Many cases of BDD have not been recorded which indicates, that it is under-diagnosed. Although there are some records, they are inadequate. The sources that have been examined provide extremely different results.

The numbers that have been recorded about this disorder's prevalence for males and females and variations between different individuals, varies from one source to another. This can be attributed to inability to correctly detect the condition by some practitioners, which leads to inadequate reports about BDD. There is therefore, inconsistency in how prevalent this condition is and how many people have it. This indicates that, there is need of emphasizing the importance of education so clinicians can know what BDD is and how they can diagnose it. This book goes a long way in helping individuals and medical experts to understand BDD and know what they can do about it. The fact that BDD is sometimes thought to be a depressive disorder or a social phobia only shows how it is mistaken with other conditions by medical practitioners. As you read on, you should apply what has been recommended to get free from this condition.

Medical professionals use Body Dysmorphic Questionnaire to be able to diagnose BDD correctly. This is a set of questions aimed at the patient which help the doctor or therapist to determine if the patient has preoccupations and if he or she is consumed with distress about an imagined flaw or a small unnoticeable real flaw. The answers given by the patient are then evaluated in accordance with the distress which affects his or her inability to function well.

The Body Dysmorphic Disorder Questionnaire has been successful in uncovering symptoms which patients are not willing to talk about. This leads to proper diagnosis and appropriate treatment. If you think you have BDD, you should be true to yourself and be genuine when completing the questionnaire. The doctor or therapist is there to help you get better. Hiding your problem will only delay your recovery. Go ahead and seek help. This is especially important if you have any of the signs and symptoms listed above.

For patients to be properly diagnosed with BDD they must fulfill the criteria stated above. In addition of medical practitioner's inability to detect BDD, diagnosis is also made difficult by patients who try to hide the disorder and often fear coming out in the open. Patients should know that, hiding it doesn't help. We encourage you to seek proper diagnosis so you can stop this condition and live a happy and meaningful life. Finally, to diagnose this condition correctly, the patient's preoccupation and obsessions must not be diagnosed other mental disorders, such as bulimia nervosa or anorexia, which are also concerns about the body image.

Chapter 2:
Steps to Take to Overcome Body Dysmorphic Disorder

The outlook for people with Body Dysmorphic Disorder is promising especially those who receive and follow-up treatment. In addition to this, those who have a strong support team have a tendency to do better in the long run. However, the most effective way to overcome this condition if you have it is to believe in yourself and your ability. You are capable of stopping this problem by facing it head on and doing what we have recommended.

Before addressing the treatment of Body Dysmorphic Disorder, it is important to understand the causes that underlie the problem. This helps you to know how to deal with this condition and it paves the way for recovery. You may have worried yourself still by now but there is hope for you. You will be able to overcome this condition if you follow what is recommended in this book.

In this chapter you will learn about the causes of Body Dysmorphic Disorder, what you can do to overcome it, the different types of treatments and the measures you can take to prevent it among other things. You will find solutions to your problems and reclaim your life back. How about that? I am sure you like it. Keep reading.

Causes of Body Dysmorphic Disorder

What causes body dysmorphic disorder? Although a lot of research has been carried out, the exact cause of BDD is not known. There are many explanations but the actual cause is not clear. What is known is that, certain biological and environmental factors may encourage its development or even trigger it.

Although the cause of BDD is not clearly known, that doesn't mean it cannot be cured. It can. This disorder, just like many other mental disorders, may develop as a result of a combination of factors. These factors include brain differences, genetic predisposition, personality traits, life experiences and other factors.

Brain differences

The brain is a major factor in the study of all mental disorders including BDD. The abnormalities in the brain structure of the sufferer or its neurochemistry may have an important role to play in the development of body dysmorphic disorder. The condition may therefore be caused by a chemical imbalance in the brain. According to research studies, the sufferer may have a problem that is caused by the malfunctioning of serotonin in the brain.

This affects the brain areas which process information about the sufferers' body appearance giving them a distorted view about themselves. This is derived from the fact that, BDD usually occurs in people who have other mental problems such as major anxiety disorders and depression. This relationship between BDD and other mental disorders supports the biological basis of this disorder. However, there are medications that stabilize serotonin levels which are used in the treatment of body dysmorphic disorder and other health problems as we shall see.

Genetic predisposition

BDD may be caused by genetic predisposition which means that, it may run in some families. Some studies have shown that, body dysmorphic disorder is likely to affect those who have relatives who have suffered from the same condition either currently or in the past, although not in all cases. The disorder is shown to be more common in people who have biological family members who also suffer or have suffered from this condition in the past.

This indicates that, there may be a gene in some families that is related to this disorder.

Environment and Life experiences

The environment and life experiences play an important role in the development and manifestation of body dysmorphic disorder. This usually happens especially if the sufferers have been involved in negative experiences about their body or their self-image. Past life experiences play a major role in the development of this disorder, because they create an environment for it. Body dysmorphic disorder may be more common in people who were teased, bullied or abused when they were children.

People who are prone to these conditions may have had:

- Life experiences of traumatic situations such as bullying and abuse.

- Emotional conflicts during childhood.

- Low self-esteem.

- Parents and other people who were influential to them as children that criticized their appearance.

- High expectations from society and peer pressure can lead to development of BDD. Today's, society has expectations that equate the physical appearance with beauty or attractiveness and value. This puts pressure that can have an impact on an individual.

Personality Traits

Another factor that might influence the development of BDD or its trigger is the personality traits of the individual.

Biological and Psychological Models

BDD is not as well researched as other body image disorders such as eating disorders but, some studies group the causes into the biological model and psychological model.

Biological Model - a person is said to have a genetic predisposition to the condition. When this person is exposed to certain life stressors like abuse or bullying, these trigger the condition. Once BDD has developed, any imbalance in the neurotransmitters within the individual such as serotonin only worsens an existing problem.

Psychological Model – Body Dysmorphic Disorder is related to the sufferers' low self-esteem. This is because they tend to judge themselves based on their physical appearance. These people may regard themselves as unattractive or ugly which are false beliefs. They may think their appearance makes them worthless which is not true.

What Can You Do?

To overcome Dysmorphic Body Disorder there are several things you can do.

Self-help care: Lifestyle and Home remedies

➢ **Always stick to your treatment plan:** Don't skip therapy sessions, even if you don't feel like going. It may be personalized therapy, family therapy or group therapy, follow instructions and do the assignments as expected. If you have a problem, feel free to discuss it with your therapist.

➢ **Take your medications** as prescribed: Stick to your regimen even when you feel better until the doctor recommends otherwise. Resist any temptation to skip taking your medications even when you feel well because symptoms may return when you stop taking them. You could also have withdrawal symptoms when you stop taking medications abruptly.

> **Learn about your condition:** This book has all the BDD resources that you need. Learning about BDD helps you to understand it and cope with it. It helps you to know what it is, how you can recognize it and how you can deal with it effectively. This motivates you to stick to your medications and therapy sessions because you understand how they help you. It paves way for full recovery.

> **Recognize the warning signs:** It is important to know how to recognize the warning signs which show the red flag when things start going wrong. We have listed these warnings in this book so you can become proactive and act before things go wrong. If you can't do it on your own, work with your doctor or therapist and learn what might trigger the symptoms or worsen the condition. Know the warning signs and make a plan about what you will do if symptoms return. It may be calling a friend or family member,

going out, listening to your favorite music or other distractions. Contact your doctor or therapist in case you notice changes in your symptoms or how you feel.

> **Be active:** Staying idle can trigger symptoms. You need to be active with physical activity and exercise. These will help you to manage stress, anxiety and depression among other symptoms. Being physically active and exercising regularly can counteract weight gain caused by effects of some psychiatric medications. Walking, swimming, jogging, running, hiking, gardening or aerobic exercises and other physical activities which you enjoy will help a lot.

> **Don't abuse drugs and alcohol:** This can trigger symptoms and make it difficult to cope with BDD and any other mental disorder. Abusing alcohol and illegal drugs can worsen your condition or interact with medications and therapy. This is counter-productive to your recovery.

> **Go for routine medical checkups:** You should attend checkups regularly as recommended by your doctor. Don't skip

visits to your family doctor so your condition can be monitored. Consult your doctor if you are feeling unwell because you may be experiencing adverse side effects to medications. You may also have another health problem that needs to be treated.

Coping and support

Coping with body dysmorphic disorder is possible as you work towards recovery, if you follow the tips we have recommended.

Tips to help you cope with Body Dysmorphic Disorder

- ➢ **Keep a journal:** It is important to keep a journal if you have BDD. Writing down what you are feeling can help you to express your fear, frustration, pain, anger, and other emotions. This relieves you of those feelings as you let them out in writing. Bolting them or hiding your feelings will only encourage them to continue. Take a notebook right away and start writing, it will make you feel better.

➤ **Don't isolate yourself:** People with BDD avoid mingling with other people. They isolate themselves. Get together with your family members and close friends. Try to participate as much as possible in social activities. Try it even if you don't feel like it.

➤ **Take good care of yourself:** You can make a difference in your life by eating a healthy diet, getting enough sleep, exercising regularly and staying physically active.

➤ **Read self-help books which have a good reputation:** Talk to your doctor or therapist and ask about good self-help books. Make sure that you read them and apply what is recommended consistently in addition to therapy. Start by reading this book to the end. You will find many things that will show you the way to full recovery.

➤ **Join a support group:** When you isolate yourself you may think you are the only one suffering from this condition. Join a support group in your area to connect with other people who are experiencing similar challenges. You will gain a lot by hearing their experiences, and how they cope with the condition. Work together as a group, it will be fun.

➢ **Stay focused on your recovery goals:** Recovery is a journey, so you should have recovery goals of how you want to go about it. Overcoming this problem is an ongoing process and therefore you should be determined and stay focused on your recovery goals. This will motivate you to keep working towards getting better, when your goals are constantly in your mind.

➢ **Practice relaxation and stress management techniques:** We know that "practice makes perfect" and this is true in anything you try to do. Learn and practice stress-reduction and relaxation techniques. Loosen up, don't be harsh on yourself. Find ways to have fun.

➢ **Avoid making major decisions:** Make decisions when your mind is clear so you can be rational.

Treatment

Treatment of BDD includes:

- Cognitive behavioral therapy (CBT)

- Medications

Many people with BDD will improve with treatment which may be a combination of medications and therapy or either of them. The specific treatment recommended will depend on how severe your condition is and how it affects your daily life. If you have mild BDD, you may be referred to a therapist for CBT which is a type of talking therapy. For more severe cases, you may be treated with SSRIs and other medications and/or more intensive CBT. Cognitive behavioral therapy trains you to recognize the irrational thoughts that you may have, and how to change your negative thinking patterns in order to change your feelings and behavior positively. You will learn through therapy how to identify the unhealthy ways of thinking, feeling and behaving, and replace them with healthy ones. The most effective treatment of BDD is believed to be a combination of CBT and SSRIs.

Cognitive Behavioral Therapy (CBT)

CBT is a type of therapy that can help you to manage your body dysmorphic disorder and other problems by changing the way you think, feel and behave. CBT is a type of psychotherapy which recognizes that thoughts, feelings and behaviors are interrelated. Thoughts affect feelings which influence actions or behaviors. You can change the way you feel and behave, by changing the way you think and this helps you to cope with your problems. CBT involves individual counseling, family therapy or group therapy. It focuses on changing your thinking (cognitive therapy) and your behavior (behavioral therapy) to overcome mental illnesses.

The goal of CBT in BDD is to correct the false beliefs about your defect or flaw which is usually minor or imagined, and to minimize your compulsive behavior. You will need to work with your therapist to agree about your therapy goals. You should practice what the therapist tells you on your own or with help i.e. stop checking yourself on the mirror excessively.

An important part of CBT that is used to treat BDD is known as graded exposure and response prevention (ERP). This is a guided type of therapy that exposes you to situations that make you obsessive and compulsive about your appearance, to help you cope better with these situations over time.

You are exposed to i.e. looking in the mirror if you avoid it or facing the public without make-up. This makes you get used to these situations so that, you can gradually change. CBT is successfully whether it is delivered to individuals, family or to a group of patients with BDD.

Cognitive behavioral therapy helps you to:

- Learn about your condition so you can understand your thoughts, feelings, moods and behavior.

- Use the knowledge you have gained, to stop negative thoughts, feelings and behaviors and view yourself realistically and in positive ways.

- Learn how to control your compulsions in healthy ways by handling these urges or rituals and routines like checking yourself in the mirror, picking on your skin etc. so that, you no longer do them automatically. This helps you to be in control of your life.

- Teach you healthy behaviors which help you to gain confidence to be able to do such things like socializing with others

Before you start therapy, you and your therapist will discuss about the type of therapy which is best for you whether personalized, family or group therapy. The discussion will also cover your goals for therapy and other issues you or your therapist may be concerned about. These will include the number of sessions you will attend and the duration of each session. You may be given some assignments to do at home between the sessions and other self-help materials. You may work as an individual or as a group and be invited to participate in group activities.

Medications

The medications used to treat Body Dysmorphic Disorder include psychiatric medications which are used for treating conditions such as depression. These are known to be effective especially SSRIs. Selective serotonin reuptake inhibitors (SSRIs) are the most common antidepressants prescribed for BDD. They ease symptoms, they are relatively safer than other medications, and have fewer side effects.

Selective Serotonin Reuptake Inhibitors (SSRIs): Medications used for the treatment of Body Dysmorphic Disorder include anti-depressants which are known as selective serotonin reuptake inhibitors (SSRIs). SSRIs are an effective type of antidepressants which increase the level of serotonin, a chemical in the brain. This chemical is used by the brain to transmit information from one brain cell to another. As we have seen earlier, serotonin changes may be responsible for development of BDD or they may trigger it. SSRIs are showing promise in the treatment of Body Dysmorphic Disorder because of their effectiveness.

SSRIs appear to be more effective than other antidepressant medications and may help to control your obsessions and repetitive behaviors. Your doctor may start you on a low dosage depending on the severity of the problem and increase the dose gradually, so you can tolerate the medications and any possible side effects.

There are different SSRIs which are available, but most doctors prescribe Fluoxetine for people with BDD. You should take your medication as prescribed although it may take a few weeks before you notice their effect. Take the medications without fail for further improvements and to prevent relapses. Your doctor may reduce the dose gradually when your symptoms are under control, to minimize any possibility of adverse withdrawal symptoms.

Other available SSRIs include:

- Citalopram (Celexa)

- Escitalopram (Lexapro)

- Paroxetine (Paxil, Pexeva)

- Sertraline (Zoloft)

Side effects of SSRIs

You may or may not experience side effects of SSRIs but it's important to know about them in case you do. However, this shouldn't worry you because most side effects fade away after the first few weeks of treatment. Talk to your doctor if you have unpleasant side effects that concern you.

Side effects of SSRIs include headaches, nausea, dizziness, insomnia, weight gain or loss, drowsiness, nervousness, restlessness, diarrheas, vomiting and agitation among others.

If you take your medication alongside your food or before bedtime (if it doesn't cause sleeplessness) you may be able to overcome nausea. Always read instructions carefully on the package insert or talk to your doctor or pharmacist about any concerns you may have. Ask questions they will be glad to answer you and help you in the process. Always know that, you are not alone in this journey, there are others who are always willing to help you cope and overcome your problems.

Other medications

There are several other medications which can be prescribed if SSRIs aren't effective in improving your condition, so, you should never give up hope. The doctor may prescribe a different type of antidepressant known as Clomipramine or others. Other treatments include antipsychotic medicines.

These are:

- Aripiprazole,

- Olanzapine

- Pimozide

These medications can either be taken alone or may be combined with Selective Serotonin Reuptake Inhibitor SSRIs. In some instances, the doctor may prescribe other medications in addition to your primary antidepressants.

Family Therapy and/or Group Therapy

Family support is very important in making any type of treatment a success. It is important that your family members understand what body dysmorphic disorder is and learn to recognize its signs and symptoms, so they can help you overcome the problem. Those who live with their parents and siblings can work as a team. At times, working towards recovery together works better because you have people to encourage you and people you are accountable to. This makes you to put more efforts to get better.

Your spouse and children can also help you cope as you strive towards recovery. We all crave to love and be loved. The first place you can easily find love is at home. Your family loves you just the way you are. In case your problems started because of the way you were treated, you don't have to hold onto this all your life, forgive and let go. This will start the healing process.

Hospitalization

In some cases, patients may be assessed and sent for psychiatric hospitalization when the symptoms are so severe. This is generally recommended when you are at risk of harming yourself like when you have suicidal thoughts or you have attempted suicide. You may also require hospitalization if you are unable to care for yourself in a proper manner.

When to see a doctor

Many people wonder at what point they should see a doctor. If you have any of the signs or symptoms of body dysmorphic disorder, which we have listed in this book, you should see your doctor, a mental health provider or any other health care professional. In most cases, people with BDD are often reluctant to seek help because they feel ashamed or embarrassed.

However, if you have BDD, there is nothing to feel ashamed or embarrassed about. It is a long-term health condition, just like many physical conditions, and it's not your fault. Seeking help is important because it's unlikely that your symptoms will improve on their own if left untreated, and they may get worse.

You should consult your GP or family doctor if you think that you may have BDD.

What to expect from the doctor

The doctor will initially, ask you a number of questions or give you a questionnaire to fill about your symptoms and how they affect your life.

These questions will probably cover the following:

- If you are specifically concerned about your physical appearance.

- Do you worry excessively about the way you look?

- Which area of your body are you concerned about?

- Do you wish you could be different?

- Do you compare yourself with others?

- When did you start worrying about your appearance?

- If your daily life is affected by the symptoms and how?

- How much time do you spend daily gazing at the mirror, skin picking or thinking about your appearance? How many hours are you concerned about your appearance in a day?

- What have you tried on your own to feel better or to overcome symptoms?

- What makes you feel worse?

- The treatments or therapy, if any, you have had, even for other ailments not necessarily BDD

- The cosmetic procedures, if any, you have you had

- If family members or friends have commented about your looks, moods or behavior.

- If you have relatives who have been diagnosed with a mental illness.

- What you hope to gain from the treatment or what your treatment goals are.

- What medications do you take? State all of them and their dosages.

- The herbs or supplements you take, if any.

- What effects do medications, herbs and supplements have on your life?

- Is it hard for you to go to school or work?

- Do you find it hard to be with family, friends and other people? Do you avoid social interactions?

If your doctor suspects that you have BDD, you may be referred to a mental health specialist to carry out further assessments and give you the appropriate treatment.

Some people who have BDD also suffer from other disorders although it is not obvious. These include eating disorders, depression, obsessive compulsive disorder (OCD) and social anxiety disorder although not all the patients do, so, you should not assume that you have these conditions unless you have received proper diagnoses. BDD can also be wrongly diagnosed as one of these conditions because of the similarity of symptoms. For example: binge eating disorder and body dysmorphic disorder are interconnected. Both BDD and OCD patients have obsessive thoughts and compulsive behaviors. People with BDD and those with social anxiety disorder, avoid social situations and social interactions.

You need to get an accurate diagnosis so you can receive appropriate treatment. You should let the doctor know the specific concerns that you have with your appearance. A medical doctor, mental health professional or a trained clinician should be able to help you. Seek help, don't hide your problems. You will be surprised to know many other people have the same problems.

You can start assessing yourself by taking a self-help test to deal with the problem as early as possible. If you have a child who is preoccupied with the appearance in a way that this interferes with his or her concentration of school work, and if you notice the symptoms stated in this book, you should talk to your family doctor or a mental health professional. Luckily, there are effective treatments to help any BDD sufferer whether young or old to live a full and productive life.

Treatment is tailored towards each individual and so, it is important to talk with your doctor to determine the best approach to your problem or your loved one's problem. Many doctors recommend a combination of treatments including therapy and medications for the best results.

Although the first doctor to talk with about your concerns may be your family doctor or a health care provider, you are likely to be referred to a mental health provider, such as a psychologist or psychiatrist, for evaluation and treatment. Treatment of body dysmorphic disorder will be difficult, if you aren't an active participant in your care. But treatment is usually successful. This will not take long after starting the treatment plan if you are willing to participate and if you are already doing what we have recommended in this book.

How to prepare for your appointment

You can manage your condition better if you actively participate in your medical care. Think about what you need and which goals you aim at with treatment. Make a list of questions you want to ask your doctor or therapist.

These may include:

- Can I get over Body Dysmorphic Disorder on my own?

- What can I do to help myself overcome this condition?

- Which self-help books can you recommend?

- How do you treat BDD?

- Are there medications that might help?

- How long will treatment take?

- Do you have any brochures or other printed materials that I can take?

- Are there any websites that you can recommend?

Don't hesitate to ask additional questions during your appointment.

Avoid the Risk Factors

To overcome BDD, you need to avoid certain risk factors as much as you can. Although the specific cause of Body Dysmorphic Disorder may not be known, there are certain risk factors which you should ensure that you avoid by all means. These factors have a tendency to increase the risk of developing or even worsening this condition or they may trigger it.

These risk factors include:

- Having biological relatives with body dysmorphic disorder (which is beyond your control but it is good to know if that is the cause of your problem)

- Having negative life experiences, such as childhood abuse, criticism and bullying

- Personality traits which lead to low self-esteem

- Societal pressure or expectations about beauty and attractiveness

- Having other psychiatric disorders, such as anxiety disorder or depression

Complications

What are the complications associated with BDD?

Complications that BDD may cause or be associated with include:

- Low self-esteem

- Depression or other mood disorders

- Difficulty attending work or school

- Social phobia and isolation

- Having no close relationships with family or friends

- Anxiety disorders such as social anxiety disorder

- Eating disorders such as Binge Eating Disorder, Bulimia nervosa and Anorexia

- Obsessive compulsive disorder (OCD)

- Unnecessary and repeated cosmetic surgery procedures such as plastic surgery

- Substance abuse i.e. alcohol or drugs

- Repeated hospitalizations

- Suicidal thoughts or attempts

Prevention

- Begin treatment as soon as you notice any signs and symptoms, before they become problems. This is very helpful. It will deter the development of this disorder.

- Those who are susceptible to get this condition can learn how to deter it by adopting healthy attitudes and behaviors as taught in CBT. They should also be realistic about their body image. This will help to prevent the development and triggering BDD.

- Those who have it already can do what is recommended in this book to prevent the condition worsening. Since this disorder is believed to develop during adolescence or during childhood, it is important to identify children and teens that are at risk of getting the disorder, so that treatment can be started early enough. This will be beneficial than treating the condition when it has already started.

- Sufferers should also receive long-term maintenance treatment in form of therapy and/or medications to prevent relapses of the symptoms.

- People who are around someone prone to BDD should provide the person with an understanding and supportive environment. This will help to decrease the severity of the symptoms and help that person cope with the disorder in a better way. This may be a parent, spouse, close friends or any other person.

Chapter 3:
What is Binge Eating Disorder?

You may have heard about Binge Eating Disorder (BED), but you don't actually know what it is, or the difference between this disorder and other eating disorders. You or your loved one could be suffering from it. Maybe that is why you are reading this book or you are concerned about a friend you would want to help. What is Binge Eating Disorder? How can you recognize it? What are the signs and symptoms? What can cause this disorder? What treatments are available and what is the prognosis of BED?

Binge eating disorder (BED) is an eating disorder which causes a person to frequently consume unusually large amounts of food and feels unable to stop eating even when full. However, binge eating is not followed by purging like in anorexia nervosa and bulimia nervosa.

The first person to describe binge eating was Albert Stunkard, a psychiatrist and researcher. That was in 1959 describing it as night eating syndrome NES.

Binge eating disorder is a very common eating disorder among adults today, although there is less media coverage and research about it, when compared with bulimia and anorexia nervosa. Binge eating disorder was only recorded as an eating disorder in 2013 on DSM-5.

Most people overeat occasionally. You may go for a second or third helping if you enjoy the food or when you are relaxed like during a holiday. We all do this and there is no problem. Even when it becomes a problem, we are able to control it before it goes out of hand. But, there are some people who eat excessively and yet they feel unable to stop eating, even when they are full. This frequent and out of control overeating may become a regular occurrence and this is where excessive eating crosses the line to become binge eating disorder.

People with binge eating disorder, may feel embarrassed about overeating and decide to stop. However, they have such a compulsion that they can't resist the urge to continue binge eating. If you are one of those people with a binge eating disorder, there is hope for you. There is treatment and therapy which can help you to overcome this problem. Better still, we will show you the steps to take to overcome this disorder once and for all. You need to stop it dead in its track and we will show you how.

Signs and Symptoms

Binge eating is the main symptom of binge eating disorder. However, you should know that, not everyone who overeats excessively has binge eating disorder. A person may have an eating problem that is not a disorder. At times one may binge eat occasionally and yet not experience the negative effects of binge eating disorder. These are usually physical, psychological, and social effects of binge eating disorder.

If you have binge eating, you may:

- Eat excessively or consume large quantities of food within a short time, even when you are not hungry. People who binge eat consume food within a specific time, like 2 hours

- Feel unable to control your eating or know that, the eating behavior is out of control. Loss of control is what makes binge eating disorder different from normal overeating whereby you are able to control the eating.

- Eat more and more food even when you are full and eat when you are not hungry.

- Eat more rapidly than is normal, especially during binge episodes

- Eat until you are uncomfortably full and feel unable to stop.

- Be obese or overweight like most people. You can still have your normal weight even when you are a binge eater.

- Feel disgusted, depressed, ashamed, upset or guilty with yourself about your eating, afterwards. Binge-eating provides only short-term relief.

- Diet or skip meals frequently between binge episodes with an intention of losing weight, which you are unlikely to lose. This is because of craving for more food, which you overeat, thus alternating dieting and overeating.

- Eat large amounts of food alone or in secret, because you feel embarrassed about how much you eat. You often binge in private because you feel guilty, ashamed or disgusted with your behavior after you finish eating.

- You don't purge or flush-up food after binge eating or use laxatives or exercise excessively, like people with bulimia. You don't feel the urge to purge the food in order to compensate for the extra calories you have gained.

- Plan binges in advance by buying special foods which you crave which may be loaded with fat and sugar.

- In some instances, people binge at night saying they don't remember what they ate because they were in a dazed state, although this is rare.

- You may be in a vicious cycle that you find hard to break. When you have binge eating disorder, you may get craving for unhealthy foods that your body doesn't need. This causes you to overeat too much fat, simple carbohydrates and food loaded with refined sugar. You may skip meals which makes you have more cravings. You may try to diet or eat less food but restricting your eating may worsen binge eating.

Binge eating episodes

Binge eating can be mild or severe. The severity of binge eating is usually determined by how often bingeing episodes occur in a week. You can have recurrent episodes of binge eating.

A binge eating episode is characterized by:-

1. Eating in a specific period of time like within a 2-hour period.

2. The amount of food eaten is definitely larger than what most people would eat normally, in the same period of time, when they are exposed to similar circumstances.

3. Lack of control and compulsive eating during the binge eating episodes. You feel that, you can't stop eating or you can't control what and how much you are eating.

These binge eating episodes are usually associated with the following:

- There is remarkable distress due to binge eating.

- Binge eating occurs, at least once a week on average, for a period of 3 months.

- There is no purging or use of laxatives like in bulimia nervosa and anorexia nervosa.

What Can Cause This Disorder?

The causes of binge-eating disorder are unknown. More research is needed to uncover the causes of binge eating disorder. But family history, biological factors, long-term dieting and psychological issues increase your risk.

Factors that can increase your risk of developing binge-eating disorder include:

Family history

A person is more likely to have binge eating disorder if the parents or siblings have or had it. Inheritable genes predispose people to this condition. This means that, heritability increases the risk of developing or triggering binge eating disorder.

There are studies that have supported the fact that, there is likely to be a genetic component running in families that is related to binge eating disorder. Research studies have shown that, binge eating tends to run in some families.

Psychological issues

Most people who have binge-eating disorder feel negative about themselves and their skills and accomplishments.

Triggers for bingeing can include:

- stress

- anxiety

- poor body image, feeling dissatisfied with your body and pressure to lose weight

- low self-esteem and lack of confidence

- feelings of anger, boredom or loneliness

Your age

People of any age can get this disorder but usually, it affects people from the late teen years or adolescence to adulthood.

Environment

Some research studies suggest that, binge eating disorder can be caused by the environment. The impact of traumatic events has a major role to play in the development of this disorder. When people experience trauma and other adverse life experiences, they tend to develop binge eating disorder. This also sets in when these negative life events occur frequently. Binge eating may not start immediately when, one experiences these adverse life events in the year prior to the onset of the development of the disorder, and that binge eating disorder was positively associated with how frequently negative events occur.

These environmental factors include:

- physical abuse and fear of abuse

- criticism about body weight

- childhood obesity

- childhood abuse

- previous stressful or traumatic events

- family-related eating disorder due to genetic predisposition

Dieting and rigid eating habits

Many people who have binge eating disorder are known to have a history of dieting. Some of them have dieted since childhood or adolescence. When people diet or they restrict the calories, this may trigger an urge to binge eat especially in those people who already suffer from low self-esteem or depression.

Previous research has focused on the relationship between body image and eating disorders, and it concludes that, binge eating might be linked to rigid dieting practices. It may begin when individuals recover from rigid eating habits. When under a strict diet that mimics the effects of starvation, the body may be preparing for a new type of behavior pattern, one that consumes a large amount of food in a relatively short period of time.

Binge eating can sometimes be caused by strict dieting, especially when meals are skipped or certain foods avoided so one can lose weight. These are unhealthy ways to lose weight and may lead to more bingeing. There is a close relationship between binge eating and restrained or rigid dieting. Rigid dieting can lead to lack of self-control when eating which makes the person to practice further rigid eating to compensate for the excess food eaten. This becomes a vicious cycle which may be hard to break unless you are determined to break it as you shall learn in this book.

Usually, binge eating is likely to happen after dieting in many instances. There are different kinds of dieting which include:

- delaying eating or avoiding eating during the day

- restricting calorie intake extremely

- avoiding certain foods such as carbohydrates or sugar which lead to cravings instead of eating healthy foods which include proteins, vegetables and fruits

There is ordinary dieting and strict dieting. Avoiding food completely after overeating makes the body weak, requiring even more food. The blood sugar level causes "spikes" when the body feels energetic. This is followed by a sudden fall in the blood sugar which makes the body weak.

Treatment and Prognosis of Binge Eating Disorder

Binge eating is treatable and most people who go through treatment and prognosis eventually get better. You can recover from binge eating disorders whether you have had it for several years or it is just starting, if you get appropriate help and support.

Diagnosis

To diagnose binge eating disorder, the doctor usually recommends an evaluation of your eating habits. You may undertake a psychological evaluation whereby you and your doctor discuss your eating habits to discover the cause of the problem. The doctor may also recommend other tests to be done to check other health conditions which are associated with this disorder. In any health problem like binge eating, there are complications that may be caused by this condition after some time, which also need to be addressed. These may include obesity and weight gain which may trigger high blood pressure, high cholesterol, Type 2 diabetes, heart disease, GERD, and sleep apnea which also need to be treated.

You may need to take the following tests:

- A physical exam

- Blood tests

- Urine tests

If you or your loved one has this disorder, you can seek help from health care professionals who include general physicians, psychologists, psychiatrists, therapists, dieticians or nutritionists, trained clinical social workers and other health professionals. In binge eating, even people who are not overweight seek help because they are concerned about their binge eating habits. Treatment can helps them to overcome their problems also.

Treatment for binge eating disorder

There are many things you can do on your own to help yourself to stop binge eating as we shall see in Chapter 5. However, it is also important to seek professional help in form of treatment and support.

The most effective treatment programs for binge eating disorder are the ones that address not just the symptoms, but they should find as much as possible, the root causes of the problem, so proper treatment can be given. Treatment also addresses the emotional triggers that cause binge eating that make it difficult for you to cope with anxiety, stress, fear, sadness, and other emotions.

Weight loss programs are also helpful if you have obesity which could endanger your health. However, you should know that, dieting can contribute to binge eating, so weight loss programs should be supervised by a professional.

The main goals for treatment include overcoming eating binges, dealing with psychological problems and losing weight only when necessary. Treatment should address psychological issues which relate to binge eating such as poor self-image, shame, guilt and other negative emotions. They should help you to feel in control of your eating.

Therapy for binge eating

Binge eating disorder can be treated with therapy successfully and recovery is possible. Therapy can teach you how to overcome compulsions and obsessions of this disorder and how to replace unhealthy habits with healthy ones.

There are 3 types of therapy that have been helpful in the treatment of binge eating disorder among others. These therapies stand out among the rest because of their effectiveness.

These are Cognitive Behavioral Therapy (CBT), Dialectical behavior therapy and Interpersonal therapy.

- **Cognitive Behavioral Therapy (CBT)** – CBT treatment has been demonstrated as a most effective type of treatment for BED and other eating disorders. It is also known to be very effective in the treatment of other conditions such as BDD as we saw earlier. CBT helps you to change your unhealthy thoughts, feelings and behaviors and replace them with healthy ones. It teaches you to cope in better ways with issues that trigger bingeing episodes. These may be negative feelings about your body or physical appearance and other issues. CBT helps you to be in control of your behavior so you are able to regulate your eating patterns and behavior. Cognitive-behavioral therapy CBT can be adopted either on its own or with other forms of treatment. This therapy focuses on changing your thoughts, feelings and behaviors, which are dysfunctional.

- **Dialectical Behavior Therapy (DBT)** – is a form of therapy that helps you to learn better skills about behavior. These improved behavioral and coping skills help you to tolerate stress which leads you to overeat. This therapy also helps you to learn how to regulates your emotions so that, you don't over-react to situations but you are able to deal with them so they don't result in undesired reactions. All these positive changes reduce your urge to binge. Dialectical behavior therapy teaches you to accept yourself, tolerate stress in better ways, and to regulate your emotions so you feel in control. Your therapist also addresses attitudes that you may have about eating, weight and shape so you can replace them with healthy attitudes about yourself. Therapy includes both individualized treatment sessions and group therapy sessions all of which are helpful.

- **Interpersonal psychotherapy** – focuses on helping you to improve your relationships with others. It addresses the problems and interpersonal issues that lead to compulsive eating. You will work with your therapist who will help you improve your interrelationships with family and friend and also your communication skills. You will learn how to develop healthier relationships with your family and friends so you can have close and stable relationships. This way, you will find that as to relate better to other people, your compulsion to binge-eat lessens your find it easier to resist those urges.

Support for binge eating disorder

There are many groups, which include formal and formal ones. Some are supervised by a therapist while others are not.

- Individualized psychological therapy – is a one-on-one therapy for individuals such as CBT. Therapy takes place between the therapist and patient.

- Group therapy – is therapy given to a group facing the same challenges. It is led by a trained therapist or volunteer. Anything that affects the group members may be discussed whether it is about binge eating or healthy eating. Members discuss about their experiences while giving and receiving advice as they support one other.

- Self-help books – read alone or with a support group and share ideas.

- Online courses – can be taken alone or as part of a support group

- Supervised self-help programs – guided by a professional by having regular contacts usually on phone.

Medications for binge eating disorder

Medications are not commonly used on their own. Since therapy has shown to be very effective in the treatment of binge eating disorder, medications are used alongside therapy only when necessary. They are included in the treatment plan as part of a comprehensive program that includes therapy, self-help groups and group support, medications and self-help steps which you can take as we shall see in Chapter 5. A number of medications may be used.

These include:

Lisdexamfetamine dimesylate (FDA approved)

Antidepressants - Selective Serotonin Reuptake Inhibitors (SSRIs) which include:

- Fluoxetine

- Sertraline

- Fluvoxamine

Anticonvulsants include:

- Topiramate

- Zonisamide

Anti-obesity drugs

Behavioral programs – for losing weight

Bariatric surgery – is preferred by some people who want to lose weight

Medications are not the priority in treating binge eating disorder because of more effective psychotherapeutic approaches, especially CBT. However there are patients who prefer to take anticonvulsant and anti-obesity drugs to lose weight in addition to therapy.

Behavioral programs for weight-loss

Weight-loss is a priority for many people with binge eating disorder who are over-weight or obese. However, restricting your diet may cause more binge eating episodes, so, these weight-loss programs should be done under medical supervision. They are also done at the appropriate time when the doctor or therapist recommends them. If this is not followed, then they may not be successful because dieting may lead to more binge eating. The medical supervision is done to make sure, that you are meeting your body's nutritional requirements. When these weight-loss programs are done alongside cognitive behavioral therapy, they are usually very effective.

Prognosis

Obesity and weight gain are some of the results of overeating. There are many health problems that arise as the consequences of binge eating disorder which affects your health and well-being. This is caused by eating excess sugar and fat which have little nutritional value.

Your food should consist of:

- Complex carbohydrates which the body releases slowly into the bloodstream unlike simple carbohydrates which cause blood sugar levels to rise and fall suddenly

- Proteins

- Fruits and vegetables

- Healthy fats

- Fiber

- Pure drinking water

- Seeds and nuts

These foods provide the body with the nutrients it requires such as vitamins and minerals to function properly and serve you better.

When you consume unhealthy foods loaded with excess unhealthy fat, sugar and salt, you become obese and your body loses the ability to fight illnesses and diseases. As a result of this you become prone to other health conditions on top of binge eating disorder because of lack of proper nutrition.

People who have obesity and they have binge eating disorder are at risk of health conditions related to obesity as we have seen earlier in this book.

This includes:

- Heart disease

- Cardiovascular disease

- High blood pressure

- High cholesterol levels

- Type 2 diabetes

- Musculoskeletal problems

- Gastrointestinal disease

- Gall-bladder problems

- Sleep apnea

These are serious problems some of which can be life threatening if proper measures are not taken. There is a lot you can do as we shall see in Chapter 5.

People who suffer from binge eating disorder are often upset about their habits and may develop anxiety, stress and depression. These problems should be treated. Binge eating also affects the quality of life which makes an individual to have difficulties with social interactions.

Treatment for binge eating disorder requires a comprehensive approach that involves a team of professionals who include medical providers such as your family doctor or general practitioners who refer you to mental health providers and nutritionists or dietitians who have experience in treating eating disorders.

When to see a doctor

There is need to see a doctor as soon as possible if you have any symptoms of binge eating disorder. Seek medical help to get help before the condition go out of hand. Binge eating disorder usually doesn't get better on its own in fact; it may worsen if it is left untreated.

First of all, you need to talk to your primary care provider or a mental health professional about your symptoms and how you feel. There are times one feels reluctant to seek medical treatment, in such cases you should talk to someone such as a family member, a close friend, a teacher or a spiritual leader about what you are going through. This should be someone you trust so you will feel free to tell him or her about your life. It should be someone who can help you to take steps towards successful treatment of this binge eating disorder. It also helps a lot to talk to someone who has the same condition if it's possible.

How you can help a loved one

When people have binge eating disorder, they tend to hide the problem which makes it hard for others to detect it even family members and close friends. If you suspect that a loved one may have this disorder, encourage him or her and offer your support. This goes a long way in helping that person cope with the symptoms and put efforts to overcome the problem. You can have an open discussion about what you have noticed. In order for that person to trust and confide in you, be honest about your concerns.

Give as much help as possible. Offer to help him or her to find a qualified doctor or a mental health provider who will recommend the treatment. Make an appointment and offer to accompany your loved one to the doctor's office. At times it can be your child, brother or sister, parent, spouse or a close friend.

Warning signs that a loved one is bingeing include finding piles of empty food packages and wrappers, cupboards and refrigerators that have been cleaned out, and hidden stashes of high-calorie or junk food which binge eaters crave for. If you suspect that your loved one has binge eating disorder, talk to the person about your concerns.

It may be a daunting task starting such a sensitive conversation with your loved ones. They may deny that they have a bingeing problem or they may feel angry that you have discovered their disorder and therefore become defensive. Don't give up because there is a chance that he or she would also want to talk about their struggle. The person may shut up at first and open up later. Just offer your compassion, support and encouragement. Be with that person through the treatment process.

What you should do when your loved ones have binge eating disorder:

- Encourage them to seek help. Urge them to seek help from a health professional. When this condition stays untreated, it gets worse that is why it is important to seek help as soon as possible.

- Provide them with your support. Listen to them attentively and avoid making judgment. Having someone who loves and cares for them may be all that they need. Show love and concern and ensure that these people know that you care. If they get relapses and slip back on the road to recovery, reassure them and keep reminding them that they can quit binge eating once and for all. Reassure them over and over again that you care about their health and their well being and that you want them to be happy and in control of their life. Tell them and you'll always be there for them.

- Set the way by being a good example to them. Eat healthy, exercise regularly, and manage your stress without using food.

- Avoid criticisms, reprimanding them or giving them lectures and issuing ultimatums. Binge eaters already feel bad about their habits already so getting upset and lecturing them will only make them feel worse. This will only make them binge eat even more to cope with stress.

- Seek help and advice for yourself if you think things are going overboard. Talk to a counselor, your family doctor or health professional. Things can be stressful, and you need support also so you can also help to your loved ones.

How to prepare for an appointment

To get ready for your appointments if you are the one who has binge eating disorder, ask a family member or a close friend to accompany you, if it is possible. The purpose is to help you remember the main points and to explain the situation in detail, from his or her own view.

What you should do

Make a list of the following before your go for an appointment:

- The symptoms you are experiencing, even those that are not related to the disorder

- All the medications you are taking including supplements and herbal treatments and their dosage

- Your food amounts and eating habit on a typical day

- Major life changes and anything else that may be causing stress

- If you have close relatives who have or had binge eating

Things to ask your doctor

- Whether binge eating disorder is a short-term or long-term condition

- The available treatments and what the doctor recommend

- Brochures and reading materials you can read

- Self-help books the doctor can recommend

Don't hesitate to ask the doctor other questions you are concerned about.

Questions to expect from the doctor

The doctor or health care provider may ask you several questions which are based on:

- Whether your eating is out of control

- How your typical daily food intake is

- If you eat unusually large quantities of food even when you are full

- If you overeat when you are full and when you are not hungry

- Whether you have tried to lose weight and how

- If you are preoccupied about food

- Whether you eat in secret

- If you feel embarrassed, ashamed or guilty about your eating

- Whether you are too concerned about your appearance and weight

- If you exercise excessively

The doctor will want to know about your compulsive eating in order to understand your eating habits and behavior to be able to schedule your treatment plan.

Other things the doctor may want to know:

- How your childhood upbringing and adolescence was.

- If you have ever been abused, bullied or criticized about body weight.

- Whether you know any relatives who have the same condition.

- Your concerns about weight, shape and size.

- If you worry excessively about your weight and hide from other people

- Whether you wish you could be different

- If you compare yourself with others

- What symptoms you experience

- If your quality of life is affected by the symptoms and how?

- What have you tried on your own to feel better or to overcome symptoms?

- The treatments or therapy you have received and whether they have been helpful

- What complications you have noted and treatments you have received for those ailments.

- Do you have other medical conditions? What treatments you had?

- What your treatments goals are and what you hope to gain from the treatment.

- The types of medications you take and their dosages.

- The herbs or dietary supplements you may be taking, if any.

- What side-effects you have experienced from the medications, herbs and supplements.

- If you avoid social interactions?

If you feel that your problems were not addressed, you can always ask the doctor for referrals to a binge eating specialist.

Chapter 4:
Other Medical Conditions Associated with Binge Eating Disorder

Binge Eating Disorder poses risks to the binge eater and it should be treated before it causes complications. That is why you should deal with this disorder and help others do the same as soon as possible before it wrecks havoc in your body. This disorder has the potential to cause long-term damage to the body organs which help in the body metabolism. There are many complications that can arise. However, appropriate and prompt treatment of binge eating disorder leads to full recovery. It also reduces the risk of these medical complications.

Other Medical Conditions

Binge eaters also develop psychological and physical problems related to binge eating. There are therefore other medical conditions associated with binge eating disorder as we shall see in this chapter. These include complications of binge eating disorder as well as other medical conditions which may develop or be triggered such as personality disorders, bulimia, anxiety disorders, major depressive disorders and irritable bowel syndrome. Some people may also develop bipolar disorder and fibromyalgia.

Complications of BED

People with BED consume large amounts of food in one sitting. This food usually consists of mainly simple carbohydrates and unhealthy fat which makes them overweight or obese. These foods don't have the nutrients the body needs to function properly. There are therefore many medical problems that arise as a result of binge eating disorder.

When a person consumes foods that are high in sugar and fat which binge eaters usually crave for and low in proteins, vitamins and minerals and other essential nutrients that the body requires to function properly, complications develop.

This may lead to many health problems which include:

- Obesity

- Type 2 diabetes

- High cholesterol

- Gallbladder problems

- Heart disease

- High blood pressure

- Digestive problems and Gastro-esophageal reflux disease (GERD)

- Sleep-related breathing disorders

- Joint pain

- Menstrual problems

If you have any of these problems, you need to seek medical help and have them treated before they become life-threatening. However, you can avoid them by eating a healthy diet, exercising regularly and following the steps recommended in this book.

Other complications that may be caused by binge-eating disorder include:

- Feeling ashamed and guilty about the uncontrollable eating habits and excess weight.

- Poor quality of life.

- Feeling bad about your life.

- Social isolation and avoiding social interactions.

- Problems functioning in school or at work.

Other Medical Conditions

Individuals with binge eating disorder have other medical conditions that are often linked with BED.

These include Body dysmorphic disorder (covered in earlier chapter), Personality disorder, Bulimia, Anxiety disorders, Major depressive disorder, Bipolar disorder, Substance use disorders, Bipolar disorder, Fibromyalgia and Irritable bowel disorder.

Personality Disorders

Personality disorders are types of mental disorders which cause individuals to differ significantly from the average person, in thoughts, perception, feelings and the way they relate with other people. The word personality means the behavioral and mental traits that make each person different from the other. When we talk about personality we mean the pattern of thinking, feeling, and behaviors that make each one of us unique.

Your personality is made up of personality traits or characteristics that you have. It is personality traits that help to distinguish you from other people. We all have a number of personality traits that are either positive or negative, but there is a general personality group which is used to describe an individual, such as extrovert or introvert among other group types. When we say that someone has a "good personality" we mean that, he or she is likeable, confident, attractive, positive, appealing, interesting and pleasant. This is how people view that person and the opposite is also true. The best thing about personality is that it can be developed. You can change negative personality traits and develop positive personality traits on your own or with therapy.

Some Positive Personality Traits

They include confidence, honesty, patience, persistence, kindness, reliability, helpfulness, intelligence, humility, obedience, conscientiousness, dependable, fairness, fearlessness, impartiality, optimism, capability, trustworthiness and integrity among others.

Some Negative Personality Traits

These include dishonesty, laziness, arrogance, cowardly, rudeness, quarrelsome, self-centered, unfriendliness, maliciousness, conceited etc.

There are many personality traits or characteristics which each society views as normal behavior. Some of these traits are in-born so they can be noticeable in childhood even in infancy, but, most of them are developed by the individual from early adolescence through adulthood. Any person who portrays an odd behavior is said to have a personality disorder. This is a collection of behaviors that differ from societal norms and expectations. Some people experience changes in how they feel while others have distorted beliefs about others which make them have odd behaviors. This can distress and upset other people. Generally these, disorders are diagnosed in most psychiatric patients and others who don't have these conditions.

Symptoms of Personality Disorders

There are different personality disorders which are grouped in Cluster A, B, and C etc. Each personality disorder has its own symptoms which are the characteristics peculiar to that disorder. In this section we shall list the generalized characteristics that are common.

Common characteristics include:

- odd behavior

- stress and depression

- becoming overwhelmed by anxiety, anger, distress, and worthlessness

- avoiding social interactions and feeling emotionally disconnected

- difficulty with relationships, especially maintaining close and stable relationships with spouse, children, work colleagues, and professional care workers

- losing contact with the reality

- difficulty coping with negative feelings which may lead to self-harm

- abusing drugs or alcohol, or taking medication drug overdoses

- threatening others although this is rare

Symptoms get worse when you have stress.

Causes of Personality Disorders

There are numerous causes of personality disorders and they vary depending on a number of factors. These include the type of personality disorder, the individual with the disorder, and the circumstances that lead to the development of the disorder.

- Genetic predispositions

- Life experiences such as trauma or abuse

- Child abuse whether physical, emotional or verbal, and neglect

Management of Personality Disorders

Many people who have personality disorders recover with time. In some instances, support is all that is required. Psychological and medical treatments are helpful although it depends on how severe the disorder is and if the patient has other medical problems. Some personality disorders improve when psychotherapy is used especially if the problem is mild or moderate. At times, therapy is combined with medications although treatment is tailored to the individual, because everyone is different and so, the responses differ.

Treatment approaches

There are many different types of treatment used:

- Personalized Therapy – this is usually in form of CBT which should be conducted by a trained therapist.

- Family Therapy – with parents, siblings or spouse.

- Group Therapy – is commonly used.

- Self-help Groups – which provide personality disorder resources and advice

- Millieu Therapy – is a group-based residential approach used to treat personality disorders i.e. therapeutic communities

- Medications –may be prescribed for the treatment of associated problems which include anxiety, depression and other problems, so that, the patient can participate in therapy. Some types of selective serotonin reuptake inhibitor (SSRI) are used. Those with mood swings may require mood-stabilizing medications. In some instances, psychiatric medications may be used.

Bulimia nervosa

Bulimia nervosa is commonly known as Bulimia. It is a common eating disorder that involves binge eating which is followed by purging. Binge eating means eating a lot of food within a short time even when the person is full, while the binge eater has no control of this behavior. In bulimia purging means attempting to get rid of the food consumed either by vomiting or taking laxatives. The sufferer may also try to lose weight by using fasting or by skipping meals, exercising excessively and taking stimulants or diuretics. Although most people with bulimia nervosa have normal weight, they still force themselves to vomit to purge the food eaten. Bulimia is associated with several mental disorders such as anxiety, depression and abuse of drugs or alcohol while in the most extreme cases, having suicidal thoughts or committing suicide.

Signs and symptoms of binge eating in Bulimia

- Lack of control over eating – the inability to stop eating is what differentiates eating disorders and normal overeating. People who overeat normally have control of their eating and they know when to stop. People with eating disorders whether bulimia, binge eating or anorexia nervosa lack this control and they continue to eat until a point where they have physical discomfort and pain.

- Eating excessive amounts of food - is common in bulimia but usually there in no obvious change in weight because of purging, excessive exercise or use of laxatives.

- Secrecy – people with Bulimia keep their eating and purging a secret. They usually eat extra food in privacy or go to the kitchen when no one is there, to eat. They go out alone for food runs.

- Food disappearance – when a binge eater is around, you may find junk food hidden somewhere, empty wrappers or food containers in the trash bin.

- Fasting or skipping meals – is common among binge eaters who alternate fasting or skipping meals with overeating to maintain their body weight or to lose weight. Where food is concerned the binge eater may want to eat all the food or nothing at all. This means that, they hardly eat normal meals like everyone else.

Purging signs and symptoms in Bulimia

- Going to the bathroom after eating – this is very common. The sufferer disappears or visits the bathroom after meals to throw up. The binge eater may run the water in the bathroom in order to disguise the sound of vomiting.

- Vomit smell – the bulimia suffers usually smell of vomit after purging. The bathroom may also smell of vomit. Although they may try to cover up the smell by using perfume, mouthwash, air freshener, mints or gum, the smell is hardly gone.

- Laxatives, stimulants, diuretics, or enemas – sufferers use these products, after they overeat to purge up food. They may also go to saunas to sweat and reduce water weight or take diet pills so they can discourage their compulsive appetite that leads them to overeat.

- Excessive exercising – is strenuous especially after overeating and may cause stress. Most of the activities done by those with bulimia include aerobics, running, skipping and other high-intensity exercises, to burn calories.

Physical signs and symptoms of Bulimia

- Scars or calluses - on the hands and knuckles caused by sticking fingers in the throat while inducing vomiting.

- Discolored teeth – caused by exposure of teeth to the stomach acid, in the purged up vomit, after throwing up. The teeth may be clear due to the destruction of enamel, yellow or ragged.

- Puffy cheeks – as a result of vomiting repeatedly.

- Patients are not underweight – men and women who have bulimia are hardly underweight. They have normal weight usually, or they are overweight but slightly. If someone is underweight while purging, this might be another type of anorexia.

- Weight fluctuations – happen frequently as a result of alternating bingeing and purging episodes.

Causes of Bulimia

There is no single cause that we can say causes bulimia. Although low self-esteem, negative body image and weight concerns about weight play a major role in causing bulimia, there are many other risk factors that are attributed to the disorder. Many people have problems dealing with their emotions and this causes not only bulimia but other eating disorders as well. Treatment especially CBT helps sufferers with confronting their fears and managing their emotions in healthy ways. When such people are anxious, stressed, depressed, sad or angry, they release these emotions by binge eating and purging. This emotional release makes them repeat the action over and over again. When all this is said and done, we can say that, bulimia is a complex emotional problem but with determination recovery is possible and we will show you how.

Major causes and risk factors for bulimia include:

- Genetic predisposition is one of the causes of bulimia, which usually runs in families. It is therefore likely that the sufferer may have a close relative with the same condition.

- Low self-esteem

- Trauma or abuse

- Stress due to major life changes

- Societal pressure and expectations about body weight

- Promotional of dieting in society's culture

- Obesity

- Parents who worry about their weight

- Psychological stress

Poor body image: is a major cause of Bulimia. Today, our culture attaches beauty and attractiveness to looks, body size and shape. This emphasis on beauty and a thin body figure, can lead people to view their bodies negatively especially women. This causes body dissatisfaction about looks, size and shape. Women are more prone to media images that portray unrealistic physical ideals about their counterparts on TV, billboards, magazines, newspapers, brochures, leaflets and others advertisements. They may hate the way they look and purge up after compulsive eating to try and look like the women on media without realizing that, these images are refined to get the attention of viewers.

Low self-esteem: there are women and men who have low self-esteem. They regard themselves as worthless, useless, and unattractive but this is only in their mind. However, if they do this repeatedly, it may put them at risk of bulimia.

The main contributors of low self-esteem are childhood abuse, depression, being a perfectionist and living in a critical home environment where parents and other family members criticize the individual.

<u>Trauma or abuse:</u> traumatic situations and being in an abusive environment can cause bulimia if one is not able to deal with it. Some people with bulimia have a history of abuse. They have higher incidences of abuse than those who don't have bulimia. They are also more likely to have parents who have problems with substance abuse whether drugs or alcohol, or they may have psychological disorders.

<u>Stress due to major life changes</u>: life can be stressful when one goes through major changes or transitions which may lead to this condition. Bulimia may therefore be triggered by:

- physical changes during adolescence

- being far away from home to attend college

- break-up of a close relationship

- separation or divorce

The person going through trauma and life changes may start bingeing and purging to cope with stress. This is a negative way to deal with these problems.

Societal pressure and expectations about body weight: people who live in societies that have high expectations about body size and shape, put a lot of pressure that makes them to develop bulimia.

Promotion of dieting in society's culture: may affect some people negatively causing them to develop bulimia.

Obesity: some people who are obese may have a negative body image and strive to lose weight in unhealthy ways by purging food.

Parents who worry about their weight: may also cause their children to do the same because they are the role models.

Psychological stress: people who encounter psychological stress due to professions or activities that put priorities about appearance are vulnerable to bulimia. These people include fashion models, actors, athletes, TV personalities, celebrities, ballet dancers and gymnasts among many others.

Diagnosis

This is based on medical history of the sufferer, although most people usually hide their binge eating and purging behavior

Management and Treatment of Bulimia

Cognitive behavioral therapy (CBT) is the main treatment of bulimia. Other treatments include SSRIs antidepressants and Tricyclic antidepressants.

- **Psychotherapy:** The psychosocial treatments for bulimia are several, but the most used therapy is Cognitive Behavioral Therapy (CBT). Others include dialectical behavior therapy and interpersonal psychotherapy. CBT can be done as personalized therapy or as group therapy. You will participate by attending therapy sessions and doing assignments between sessions. It involves teaching the sufferers to challenge their thinking and behaviors to influence how they feel. They are taught to challenge their automatic thoughts and engage in positive behaviors. In CBT people are encouraged to avoid emotional changes that make them binge and purge. They identify the emotions that make them binge and purge. They record how much food they consume and when they purge so that they avoid emotional changes that trigger bulimia episodes. CBT is effective and most of the people who use it become symptom-free. However, for it to be effective, the sufferers must participate.

- **Family Based Treatment (FBT)** – tends to be more effective for younger adolescents with eating disorders who still need guidance and guidance at that stage in their lives, from their families. Young adolescents may not realize the consequences of bulimia at that stage, so they lack the will power and motivation to change, which is necessary for CBT to become effective. That is why FBT is more helpful for them so their families intervene and support them. The teens' families are likely to support them by getting involved in their food choices and behaviors. They take the initiative to put more control at the beginning and teens take control gradually when they can practice healthy eating habits.

- **Medications:** SSRI antidepressants have shown benefits in the treatment of bulimia. These include Fluoxetine (FDA approved), Sertraline and Topiramate although it has more side effects.

Some of the positive outcomes of treatments include:

- There is an increase in abstinence from binge eating

- There is a decrease of obsessive behavior and preoccupations to lose weight and regain shape

- There are less severe psychiatric signs and symptoms

- People have a desire to counter any effects of their binge eating

- There is improved social functioning and lower relapse rates

Steps to Bulimia recovery

May be you have been living with bulimia for quite a while and you have been concealing your bingeing and purging behavior, you should know that, there is hope for you. Feeling ashamed about what you have been doing is human nature. You probably binge alone. You may have tried to control your bingeing and purging but failed. You may have been consuming foods like doughnuts and other snacks and hiding the wrappers or you may have been replacing the food so your family and friends won't notice. You may be shopping at different places so no one can know you have a problem. But there is no way you can hide from people who care about you. Despite your secret life, your family and close friends might already know something is wrong. You need to take the following steps because bulimia is curable.

Admit that you have a problem: This is where you start your recovery. Unless you admit that you have a problem, you may not realize you need to do something about it. Those who are closest to you may have tried to help you without success. It all starts with you. Don't fight this, accept it and start working towards recovery. Maybe you have been waiting for that moment when life will get back to the way it used to be and hoping that one day life will be better. You may have talked to your GP about other issues but not about bulimia. You may have convinced yourself that if only you can lose more weight you can control what you eat and you will finally feel better. The first step towards bulimia recovery is to admit that you have a distorted relationship with food and your compulsive eating is out of control.

- **Talk to someone**: you may find talking to someone about your problems hard but it is the easiest thing to do. It doesn't matter whether you have been keeping your bulimia a guided secret even from your close family members and your best friends for a long time, the time to talk about it is now. Talk to someone who can listen to you without being judgmental. Talk about what you're been going through. You may feel ashamed about yourself, guilty or afraid of what people will think but someone who cares will not mind about all that. Know that you are not alone. Your parents, siblings, spouse, children, close relatives and friends care about you and they want the best for you. Find someone who walk with you through the recovery process and support you as you works toward getting better.

- **Break the vicious cycle**: bulimia is a mental disorder which causes people to get into a vicious cycle, of compulsive overeating, purging, and overeating again. Breaking the vicious cycle is also known as breaking the habit. You need to stop the vicious cycle of bingeing and purging and restore normal eating patterns. Once you understand this and you believe that you can, then, you start trying. This way, you start learning how to monitor your eating habits and avoiding anything that can trigger binges. Find ways to deal with stress, fear and anxiety that doesn't involve eating food

- **Eat regular meals**: eat what you would normally eat. This is to help you minimize food cravings. Hold the food and preoccupy yourself with other things like listening to music, watching your favorite movie, reading or calling a friend on phone to distract your urge to purge.

- **Don't skip treatment**: CBT helps you to change unhealthy thoughts and patterns. Don't skip sessions even when you don't feel like going. Therapy helps you to identify and change any beliefs about your body weight, shape and dieting which are dysfunctional replacing them with healthy ones. You change your attitudes about eating and self-worth which has nothing to do with weight. These are just stereotypes that people believe and they end up haunting their lives.

- **Solve emotional issues**: some people have emotional issues they have carried from childhood. Others are caused by spouses and close friends. The best thing is to let go. They are only hurting you not them. Don't carry the baggage. Face your emotional issues. Therapy will help you to confront and tackle low self-esteem, relationship issues, anxiety and depression and feelings of loneliness and isolation that are the underlying causes of bulimia and other problems.

- **Understand yourself**: what is it that triggers bingeing and purging? Avoid people, foods, places, situations and activities that trigger the problem. You may find that these tempt you to binge or purge and before you know it, you are already doing it.

- **Seek help**: There are trained professionals who can help you eat normally and regain your health as well as learn healthy eating habits. They can also help you to deal with stress and develop healthy attitudes about your body and how to handle food. You will realize that, overeating and purge will not improve your poor body image and low self-esteem.

Anxiety disorders

Anxiety disorders are mental disorders whereby the sufferer has extreme fear and anxiety. This is not the normal fear and anxiety we all go through when faced with flight-or-fight situations. It is an extreme feeling that the individual is unable to control. Fear is a normal reaction to current situations and events, while anxiety is worrying about future situations and events. However, when an individual regularly suffers from extreme fear and anxiety that it adversely affects his or her life, then that is anxiety disorder. These extreme feelings may cause several symptoms.

Symptoms of Anxiety Disorders

Anxiety disorders are a group of related conditions, and each with unique symptoms. However, all anxiety disorders have one thing in common, a persistent, excessive fear or worry in usual situations that are not threatening.

People can have one or more of the following symptoms:

- Headaches and fatigue

- Fear and nervousness

- Feeling apprehensive

- Feeling tense, restless or irritable

- Anticipating the worst and watching expectantly for any signs of danger

- Panicking, heart pounding, and shortness of breath

- Sweating, trembling or shaking and twitches

- Frequent urination

- An upset stomach and diarrhea

There are several anxiety disorders which include:

- Generalized anxiety disorder

- Panic disorder

- Social anxiety disorder

- Specific phobia

- Agoraphobia

- Separation anxiety disorder

- Substance/medication-induced anxiety disorder

Anxiety is a common characteristic in all anxiety disorders although each may have varying characteristics and symptoms.

Anxiety disorders often occur together with other mental disorders such as eating disorders, personality disorders, bipolar disorder and major depressive disorder. You can see how all these conditions are related.

Causes of Anxiety Disorders

Scientists believe that many factors combine to cause anxiety disorders:

- Genetics - play an important role in the developments of anxiety disorder with some families having more people who have anxiety disorder. Research studies support that, anxiety disorders run in some families where they are prevalent.

- Stress - is a strong risk factor in the development of anxiety disorder. A person who goes through a stressful or traumatic situation or event such as death of a loved one, abuse, prolonged illness or violence may develop an anxiety disorder.

- Smoking – is a risk factor.

- Caffeine – contributes to development or triggering anxiety disorder.

- Withdrawal from drugs including medications

Treatment of Anxiety Disorders

Since each anxiety disorder has its own set of symptoms, there are different types of treatments that your doctor, therapist or mental health professional may recommend.

Treatment options include:

- Lifestyle changes

- Therapy

- Medications

Medications are usually recommended only after trying other treatments which are found to be ineffective. Anxiety disorders are more common in females than in males and usually begin during childhood.

Lifestyle changes

Smoking and taking caffeine may aggravate anxiety disorders so you should avoid them. Stopping these habits tends to have more benefits on the individual, than taking medications.

Stress and relaxation techniques, regular exercise and coming-off or reducing caffeine are often useful in treating anxiety.

Therapy

CBT is an effective treatment for anxiety disorders. CBT has two main components, cognitive and behavioral as the name indicates. When someone has anxiety disorders, the cognitive component can help people to question their unrealistic or distorted beliefs. The behavioral component changes their reactions to situations and events that trigger anxiety.

Computer-based Behavioral Therapy is carried out via the internet and it is equally effective.

Medications

Medications are indicated only if other measures have not been found to be effective or a person is not interested in trying them.

- SSRIs are recommended as first-line agents.

- Benzodiazepines as second-line drugs for short-term use

- MOIs i.e. tranylcypromine, phenelzine are effective treatments mainly used when there is resistance to other drugs.

- Pregablin is also effective

SSRIs are commonly used to treat children and adolescents. Other antidepressants include SNRIs and Tricyclic antidepressants.

Older adults, who have other physical problems are more likely to have adverse side-effects from these medications, so, more care should be taken while treating them.

Irritable Bowel Syndrome (IBS)

Irritable bowel syndrome affects the digestive system and it can be a long-term problem.

Main symptoms of IBS

- abdominal pain and stomach cramps

- changes in bowel habits such as bloating, constipation and diarrhea

- flatulence/excessive wind

- experiencing an urgent need to visit the toilet more than usual

- feeling like you haven't emptied your bowels fully, after relieving yourself

- passing mucus with stool

Other symptoms related to IBS include:

- lack of energy/lethargy

- feeling sickly

- backache

- bladder problems

- anxiety and depression due to the impact IBS symptoms have on the individual

The severity of symptoms varies from one person to another. Some people have mild to moderate IBS while in others it is so severe. The symptoms can come and go or they may be long-term problems. But, even when the condition is long-term, it may improve with time after treatment.

Causes of IBS

The exact cause of IBS may be unknown, but sensitivity of the gut and digestive problems are known to cause this condition. These problems cause bloating, constipation and diarrhea because of the way food passes through the gut. It may move too quicker or slower than it normally does and these changes in the gut cause problems. Stress may also predispose people to IBS.

Treatment of IBS

If you have IBS, you can manage the symptoms by making diet and lifestyle changes.

Diet and Lifestyle changes include:

- identifying and avoiding foods that trigger the symptoms

- increasing fiber in the diet

- exercising regularly

- reducing your stress levels

Medications are prescribed to treat anxiety, stress and depression as well as other symptoms.

Managing IBS

IBS is an unpredictable condition, at times, people can go for several months without experiencing symptoms, while other times they can have flare-up. People with IBS may experience abdominal pain, anxiety, stress or depression, which affect your daily life. If you suspect that you have this condition, talk to your doctor so you can receive treatment for the symptoms such as anxiety and depression which rarely improve without the appropriate treatment. Your doctor may recommend treatments such as CBT or antidepressants to help you manage this condition. When you receive appropriate treatment, you can live a normal active life.

Major depressive disorder

Major **depressive disorder** (**MDD**) has many other names. It is also known as **clinical depression**, **major depression** and **recurrent depression**. MDD is a mental disorder that causes the patient to have persistent sadness and low moods which are followed by low self-esteem and having no pleasure or interest in enjoyable activities which other people normally enjoy. Although people use the term depression to mean low moods, major depressive disorder is a condition that disables the sufferer and may lead to emotional and physical problems which affect his or her family, school and work life, eating and sleeping patterns and general health in many adverse ways. In the most extreme cases these peoples have suicidal thoughts or they commit suicide if the disorder isn't treated.

If you have depression, it affects how you feel, think and behave and that is why CBT is an effective and safe way of dealing with this disorder. You may be unable to do normal day-to-day activities, and you may feel as if life is worthless.

Depression usually requires long-term treatment. However, most people with depression feel better after receiving treatment so you should always have hope.

Signs and Symptoms of Major Depressive Disorder

- Having low moods regularly

- Feeling sad, unhappy and worthless persistently

- Loss of interest in normal activities

- Feeling angry, irritable or frustrated

- Lack of concentration

- Feeling worthless or guilty, blaming yourself or others for past failures

- Sleep disturbances either too much sleep or insomnia

- Feeling too tired and having no energy, requiring extra effort to do small tasks

- Being anxious, agitated or restless

- Having a change in appetite either increased or reduced appetite

- Thinking, speaking and moving slowly

- Having trouble making even simple decisions or remembering things

- Physical problems i.e. headaches or back pain which can't be explained

- Suicidal thoughts, attempts or committing suicide in the most severe cases

Lifestyle and home remedies for depression

Depression generally isn't a disorder that you can treat on your own. But in addition to professional treatment, there are several things you can do to relieve the symptoms and feel better.

These self-care steps can help:

- **Stick to your treatment plan**: Don't skip psychotherapy sessions or appointments. Even if you're feeling well, don't skip your medications. If you stop, depression symptoms may come back, and you could also experience withdrawal symptoms.

- **Learn about depression**: Learning about your condition empowers you and motivates you to stick to your treatment plan. Encourage your family to learn about depression to be able to help and support you.

- **Pay attention to warning signs**: Know the warning signs and be proactive so you don't over-react. Discuss with your doctor or therapist to know what triggers your symptoms and make a plan so you know what to do if your symptoms get worse. If you notice changes in the way you feel then contact your doctor or therapist. Ask your family members or close friends to help you watch for the warning signs so you can take appropriate measures.

- **Exercise regularly**: Physical activity reduces depression symptoms. Consider walking, jogging, swimming and gardening or take up another activity that you enjoy.

- **Avoid alcohol and illegal drugs**: It may seem like alcohol or drugs lessen depression symptoms, but in the long run they generally worsen symptoms and make depression harder to treat. Talk with your doctor or therapist if you need help with alcohol or substance abuse.

- **Get plenty of sleep**: Sleeping well is important for both your physical and mental well-being. If you're having trouble sleeping, talk to your doctor about what you can do.

Psychotherapy

Psychotherapy is known in other terms as talk therapy, psychosocial therapy or counseling. Psychotherapy has been successful in the treatment of depression either on its own or with medications. It treats depression by encouraging patients to talk about their condition, symptoms and other related issues with mental health providers. There are different types of psychotherapy which have been effective in the treatment of depression.

These include:

- Cognitive behavioral therapy (CBT)

- Dialectical behavior therapy

- Interpersonal therapy

- Acceptance and commitment therapy

- Mindfulness techniques.

Therapy can help you in:

- Identifying negative thoughts, beliefs, feeling and behaviors and replacing them with healthy and positive ones.

- Adjusting to any crisis you may be facing and solving difficult situations without over-reacting to them.

- Exploring your interpersonal relationships and developing positive interactions with other people

- Identifying triggers to depression and changing your behaviors to avoid these triggers

- Being able to identify warning signs so you can be aware of them and act before the occur

- Developing skills to help you cope and solve your problems in better ways

- Being satisfied with your life and gaining control in order to ease symptoms of depression i.e. unworthiness, hopelessness and anger

- Managing distress and stress that are caused by challenges in life, using healthier methods

- Learning how to set realistic goals and having realistic expectations from your life

Medications

Medications are also effective especially for the most severely depressed. If you have major depressive disorder, or you have a loved one with this condition, consult a mental health provider immediately. You can also ask for referrals from your family doctor or health care provider. Depression is a major disorder that will not heal on its own. Hospitalization may be necessary where the patients are a risk of harm to themselves or others and where they aren't able to care for themselves.

Selective serotonin reuptake inhibitors (SSRIs):

Doctors start by prescribing an SSRI because they are safer and generally cause fewer side effects than other antidepressants.

SSRIs include:

- Fluoxetine (Prozac)

- Paroxetine (Paxil)

- Sertraline (Zoloft)

- Citalopram (Celexa)

- Escitalopram (Lexapro)

Serotonin and norepinephrine reuptake inhibitors (SNRIs):

- Duloxetine (Cymbalta)

- venlafaxine (Effexor XR)

- desvenlafaxine (Pristiq)

Norepinephrine and dopamine reuptake inhibitors (NDRIs):

- Bupropion (Wellbutrin)

Atypical antidepressants:

- Trazodone

- Mirtazapine (Remeron)

- Vilazodone (Viibryd)

Other medical conditions associated with binge eating disorder are bipolar disorder and fibromyalgia.

Bipolar disorder

Bipolar disorder is a mental disorder which causes people to have elevated moods followed by depressive moods. The elevated moods are referred to as mania and the depressive moods are known as depressive. During mania the person is so happy and energetic as well as easily irritable. At this time, the person can make poor decisions without thinking about what the consequences will be. This is followed by depression when the person usually cries, is in low moods and usually has negative views about life. It during this depressive period that the individual may have suicidal thoughts or self-harm, and is also likely to abuse drugs or alcohol. This includes taking excess medications.

Causes of bipolar disorder

Genetic predispositions and environmental factors have a major role to play in causing bipolar disorder. These causes genes that cause this disorder in some families and environmental factors which include stress and childhood abuse.

Treatment of bipolar disorder

Treatment usually includes therapy and medications. Psychotherapy is effective and it can be given on its own or combined with medications. The commonly used medications are mood stabilizers as well as antipsychotics. Mood stabilizers include medicines such as lithium, anticonvulsants and other types. The side-effects of medications should be watched as well as other medical conditions such as heart disease which should be treated. Antidepressants may be stopped when someone during mania periods and continued during depressive periods. During these times, mood stabilizers can also be used. A person may have severe behavioral issues which can be managed with benzodiazepines and antipsychotics. In some instances, electroconvulsive therapy can be beneficial when patients don't respond to other types of treatments. Withdrawal from medications should be done slowly to avoid withdrawal symptoms from treatments.

Fibromyalgia

Fibromyalgia (**FM**) is another medical condition which causes chronic pain which is widespread through the body and other symptoms.

Symptoms include:

- Chronic pain

- Tiredness

- Joint pain and stiffness

- Sleep disturbances

- Bladder and bowel problems

- Difficulty swallowing food

- Numbness and tingling etc.

Causes of fibromyalgia include:

- Genetic predisposition

- Psychological problems

- Neurobiological causes

- Environmental factors

Chapter 5:
Can You Do Anything About Binge Eating Disorder?

Yes, you can.

There are many times we overeat and take an extra helping whether it is during the holidays, a Thanksgiving dinner or during the Christmas season. From time to time, we feel full and yet we reach out for another helping or dessert. This is not binge eating disorder. People who are binge eaters overeat frequently and they are unable to control it. They use food to cope with their stress, anxiety and other negative emotions but they even feel worse afterwards instead of feeling better. Binge eating may lead to shame and guilt which worsens the situation if the sufferer is unable to deal with it. Fortunately, you can overcome binge eating and this is the best thing you want to hear. It is curable and you don't have to go on with it. You can find your way to full recovery and we will show you how if you keep reading.

When you are a binge eater, it is important to know the truth that, binge eating is treatable. You may be in a vicious cycle, but there is hope for you and there is so much that you can do. In this chapter, you will find the solution to your problem. You may not be the one with binge eating disorder. It may be a loved one or a friend. Let them know that it is curable. If you are the one who is binge eating, whether it has started recently or many years ago, don't worry because you can stop it by following what is recommended in this book. You can also recommend the book to others who have the same or similar disorders. With the right help and support, you can learn to control your eating and develop a healthy relationship with food.

Steps to Take to Help with the disorder

Stick to your treatment plan

Follow the treatment plan by taking your medications as planned and don't skip therapy sessions even when you think you are well. Stick to your meal plan strictly and don't allow setbacks to hold you back. Any change in your treatment plan can derail your achievements and waste your efforts and the milestones you have gained. Determination and focusing on your goals will keep you strong.

Eat your breakfast

Many people who have Binge Eating Disorder usually skip their breakfast expecting that this will help. If you don't eat breakfast, you will be tempted to eat more, later in the day. You will likely consume foods with higher calories to compensate for breakfast. Eat a healthy breakfast and start your day feeling strong. This way, you may avoid bingeing during the day.

Eat three meals a day

Plan and eat 3 meals in a day and healthy snacks in a day. Eat a balanced diet and enjoy fresh fruits and veggies, seeds and nuts which are rich in vitamins and minerals. If you miss any of these meals you start craving for unhealthy foods.

Consume highly nutritious foods

If you are a binge eater you may be eating a lot of food during binge episodes which may not be nutritious. You need to consume foods that supply all the nutrients the body needs. Eat a balanced diet that includes plenty of fresh fruits and vegetables, dietary fiber, proteins and not just carbohydrates and fats. Ask the doctor if you need to take vitamin and mineral supplements. Buy organic foods if you can.

Avoid unsupervised dieting

Dieting is one of the causes of Binge Eating Disorder. Trying to diet and avoiding eating, can trigger binge episodes. This can lead you to overeat and then to alternate with dieting which causes more bingeing. This is a vicious cycle that you need to break and it requires hard work. However, you can break it if you are determined. You may fail a few times since your body may take long to adjust but keep trying and you will achieve what you have set to do with time. A journey of a thousand miles starts with the first step. Talk with your doctor to recommend appropriate strategies for weight management and follow the advice given. Avoid dieting unless the doctor or therapist recommends it as part of the treatment which should be supervised by your doctor.

Don't Diet

If you are overweight or obese you might think that, going on a diet will help you to lose weight. Diet usually backfires for many people who have gained weight. Don't diet. If you have Binge Eating Disorder, dieting can make you prone to overeating. When you restrict your body from certain foods or calories in order to lose weight, you psychologically feel deprived. These psychological changes and the chemical changes that take place in your system make the body to demand food and this encourages you to keep on bingeing.

When you binge you feel better in the short term, but later, you start beating yourself for doing it. This may stress you or make you anxious, you may also avoid eating to make up for what you overate. When you don't eat enough, the vicious cycle continues only for you to binge again. During treatment, your doctor or therapist will encourage you not to diet without supervision even after you get better. This is because dieting triggers an urge to continue bingeing in many cases. That is why you are never advised to slim by dietitians and doctors who treat your Binge Eating Disorder. You lose weight by stopping to binge. You don't lose weight to stop bingeing it's vice versa.

Be active

Ask your health care provider what kind of physical activity is appropriate for you, especially if you have health problems related to being overweight.

Arrange your environment

Availability of certain foods can trigger binges for some people. Keep tempting binge foods out of your home or limit your exposure to those foods as best you can.

Stay connected

Keep in touch with family members and don't isolate yourself from them because they care about you. Your family members whether they are your parents, siblings, spouse or children and friends want to see you get healthy. Understand that they love you and they have your best interests at heart. They would want you to be happy.

Open up about your problems

Talk to a close relative or a friend you trust about your problems. Don't hide and think people will think negatively about you. This is not the case, they will be willing to help you overcome your problems and live a happy life. Take a step and talk to someone.

Don't eat secretly

Seek help for any underlying problems like stress and depression because they may cause you to eat in order to feel good but this is only a temporary relief. Find a permanent solution instead of using food.

Try to eat slowly

You are likely to overeat if you eat quickly. Try to eat slowly and enjoy your food. Remind yourself that you don't want to overeat over and over again.

Practice and keep practicing

There is nothing of value that comes easily. You may have heard "No pain no gain". Practice healthy eating habits and keep practicing. Don't give up however hard it becomes. Focus on your recovery goals and reward yourself for small achievements but not with food.

Find ways to manage stress

Overcome stress by exercising, using stress relaxation strategies, and practicing deep-breathing exercises. Help someone who needs you and by doing so you will feel happy and fulfilled. Do voluntary work if you can and this will divert your attention from yourself to others.

Avoid food temptations

You can do this by getting rid of junk foods and other unhealthy snacks in the fridge, shelves and cupboards, where you easily reach them when you need to binge eat. Keep a bowl of healthy seeds and nuts where you usually reach out for junk foods. Drink pure drinking water instead of packaged and bottled soda or juice. Buy fresh fruits and vegetables which you can eat anytime you feel like bingeing.

Distract yourself when bored

Some people take snacks when they are bored, if you are one of them, find ways to distract yourself from boredom. Do some household chores, gardening or painting, take a walk, read a book, listen to your favorite music or call a friend on phone. Take up a hobby that you enjoy.

Get enough sleep

Take a nap in the afternoon if you are tired instead of snacking or go to bed earlier than usual if staying late at night, makes you look around for something to eat. Get enough sleep at night because if you don't, you might be stressed which encourages bingeing.

Learn to listen to your body

Our bodies speak to us in many ways. There is a time your body tells you that you are physically hungry and when it tells you that you are emotionally hungry. Deal with your emotions and avoid eating to get comfort. Eat during meal times or when you are hungry. Stop eating when you feel full. If you have cravings distract them, eat healthy foods like fruits and veggies or give yourself time for the cravings to pass.

Join a support group

If you have binge eating disorder, you and your family may find support groups helpful to provide you with encouragement, togetherness, hope and advice on how to cope with the disorder. Support group members can understand what you're going through because they've been there themselves. You need to join a support group to help you cope with the stress of your disorder. Listening to the experiences of other binge eaters can ease your pain. There is nothing as relieving as knowing that you are not alone in your journey. Ask your doctor or therapist about support groups in your area.

Reinvent your meals

Many people look forward to mealtimes when they can enjoy their favorite foods. Unfortunately, this can be a challenging time for people with binge eating disorder. Furthermore, their binges are also more likely to happen between meals when they eat snacks. You should look at food in a new way. Focus on nutritious foods that nourish your body and keep you healthy. At times, eating unhealthy foods makes your body crave for more of those foods because it's not getting the right nutrients.

Tackle it together

This condition is likely to put a strain on your family and relationships. Talking about it usually helps by tackling it together although a single conversation will not solve the problem. The best place to talk about binge eating disorder and find solutions is in family therapy especially when your child or teen has this condition. When there is open dialogue in family therapy sessions, it encourages you and your child to have open conversations at home. Make proper food choices and lead by example if you are a parent.

If your loved one is an adult, he or she may receive individual therapy, and then you can help by discussing things openly at home. Be genuine to each other to avoid conflicts. Listening with an aim to understand helps your loved one gain trust. Don't always talk about food or focus on eating every time you are together. You can go out, take a walk, visit the museum or watch a movie together. Encourage your loved one to follow the steps we have recommended. If he or she does this, the problem will start disappearing.

Family members and caregivers need to take care of themselves also, as we have seen earlier. Seek help and support when you are caring for a loved one. It may be straining but working together makes you achieve goals much faster because you are using the power of synergy. What you can both achieve together is more than what you can achieve as individuals when it is combined.

Tips to help you cope with Binge Eating Disorder

Living with an eating disorder is especially difficult because you have to deal with food on a daily basis.

Get easy with yourself

Don't beat yourself up. Feeling guilty about your eating habits and self-criticism will not help. They'll only derail your efforts to get better. Forgive yourself if you relapse but don't give up, keep trying.

Have a plan of action

Identify situations that may trigger destructive eating behavior so you can develop a plan of action to deal with them.

Role models

Look for people who can be your role models to help lift your self-esteem. Some of the models you see on TV or magazines have unrealistic bodies because of photo shooting and make ups. Look for positive role models who can influence your life positively.

Confide in someone you trust

Try to find a trusted relative or friend whom you can talk with about what's going on.

Get someone to be accountable to

Find someone who can partner with you against binge eating. This is someone you can call for support when you feel like bingeing.

Keep a journal

Consider keeping a journal about your feelings and behaviors. This can help to make you more aware of your feelings and actions so you can influence them I the right direction.

Develop healthy relationships with food

People who have compulsive eating behavior have distorted relationships with food. Develop a healthier relationship with food by eating for your nutritional needs, instead of emotional needs.

Seek Support

At times it's hard to overcome bingeing on your own. That is why you need to seek support especially from family and friends. Spend time with people who have healthy eating habits so they can influence you positively. Seek company of family members and close friends who will encourage you to eat healthy. Avoid those people who criticize you about your eating habits or your weight.

Manage stress in a healthy way

There are many healthy ways that you can use to manage stress. When some people feel stressed they overeat. This is not the right way to cope with stress. Although you may feel less stressed when you binge, it is only in the short term. Stress is part of life and you can't avoid it altogether. The healthy way to help you to relax is to practice things like exercise, calling a friend or doing something you enjoy. Take a walk, watch your favorite movie, listen to music or talk to someone. All these will make you feel better and divert your mind from bingeing.

Pause

When you are faced with a challenge that urges you to overeat, the best thing is to pause for a while and ask yourself whether you are hungry. At times, you may just want to eat because that is what your mind is focusing on. Challenge such thoughts and don't allow them to control you. You can change your behavior by practicing what you have learnt in cognitive behavioral therapy (CBT).

Change your environment

Binge eating is a behavior that puts you on autopilot when you start. You hardly realize what you are doing. Change your environment by changing the chair you usually sit on, your position or the room. If you are in the kitchen and you feel like bingeing, go to another room or take a walk and see if this will help you to make better eating decisions.

Seek Treatment

Treatment for binge eating disorder mainly involves counseling and at times medications.

The treatment goals are to help you:

- Develop a positive image about yourself and your body.

- Reduce the number of eating binges and eventually overcome the disorder.

- Develop healthy eating habits.

- Deal with the shame or guilt caused by the eating disorder.

- Get treatment for other conditions such as stress, depression, anxiety, and other underlying problems.

Most of the people with binge eating disorder require treatment but many of them don't seek treatment. They deny that they have the problem if someone tells them about their concerns while others keep it as a secret. They may talk to the doctor about obesity and their concerns about weight but fail to open up about bingeing. These people may also join weight-loss programs for weight management, in order to lose weight, but avoid seeking treatment for binge eating disorder. They may also avoid seeking treatment for mental health problems that are related to this disorder. That is why they need support from family members and friends to encourage them to seek treatment.

Counseling

Counseling is an effective treatment for binge eating disorder, in fact, more effective than medications.

- Cognitive behavioral therapy – can help you control the compulsion or urge to binge eat. This is especially helpful when it is combined with nutritional counseling and a supervised weight-loss program. Therapy will help you to learn how to eat a balanced diet so you can hasten recovery. Regular eating during mealtimes with no dieting, can help reduce your binge eating.

- Interpersonal therapy – can help you develop healthy relationships and reduce your emotional reactions which cause some of the symptoms of binge eating.

- Dialectical behavior therapy – focuses on helping you to develop skills that help you to manage your emotions better. This helps to reduce stress-related binge eating. We all deal with stress differently when we are faced with life's challenges. You may become emotional which makes you to binge when you are stressed. If you are like that, therapy can help you cope better with life's challenges which make you stressed as well as manage your emotions instead of binge eating.

Medications

The treatment for binge eating disorder includes antidepressants when the underlying problem is depression. These may be used to reduce binge eating episodes and in the treatment of related depression or anxiety.

Talk With Your Doctor

Binge eating disorder is treatable and it can be cured, if you get proper treatment.

When to contact your health care provider

Seek help if you think you have binge eating disorder. Check the symptoms we have listed and call your health care provider.

Treatment of mental health takes priority because this condition starts as a mental disorder before it creates physical problems like obesity and its complications. Binge eating disorder is known to be a complex condition which not only affects the body but also the brain. As we have seen negative thoughts, feelings and behaviors trigger overeating. You find yourself with obsessions and compulsions that lead you to binge eat. This is therefore more of a psychological problem making you to eat too much and to continue eating even when you are full. This causes you to gain a lot of weight and become obese which are physical problems which cause other medical problems. One thing leads to another.

Treatment should focus more on mental health, rather than weight loss. Weight gain and obesity are the effects of this mental problem, not the causes of binge eating disorder. It therefore may not help to address weight-loss without addressing the mental causes of this disorder. The main aim of treatment is to uncover why you binge eat and replacing the negative behaviors, emotions and thoughts with positive ones to help you get better.

Combining therapy with supervised weight-loss programs is very effective.

Start the conversation

Binge eating disorder can be a very sensitive issue for most people you may not feel comfortable talking about it. It is important to talk to your family doctor or health care provider. You may have hidden this problem for a long time in previous visits but the fact that you tried bringing the issue up before, but it didn't work out, doesn't mean it is impossible.

Maybe the conversation didn't take-off or it started but it didn't go as you had hoped. This should not deter you from starting a conversation with your doctor again. Now that you know how important opening up and having treatment are, after reading this book, you should take the initiative to start the conversation.

There is more awareness about binge eating disorder today, so, doctors and other health care providers have information about this medical condition, which can help you. That is why you should feel confident about having this conversation with your doctor because it will be to your benefit. You should start the conversation whether you have tried to talk about it before or not. You should open up even if it is your first time to have a discussion about BED. This is because your health is very important not only to yourself but to others as well.

Start the conversation by talking about what is going on in your life specifically about your eating. The doctor can help you by providing you with the support you require. You may share about specific bingeing episodes which you had. Talk about how long the bingeing episodes were, how long you have been having these episodes, how much food you usually consume, what is happening in your life and how you feel during and after overeating. The discussions you will have with your doctor or therapist and in some cases mental health provider will help to uncover the cause of the problem and the symptoms you experience so that an appropriate treatment plan can be arranged.

Although you may not feel comfortable at first, you will find it easier as you open up. Remember that, there are many people who suffer from the same condition who are having similar conversations with their health care providers looking for help.

List down the symptoms you have been experiencing before you go for your appointment. This will help your health care provider to understand about the condition whether you choose to visit your family doctor or a specialist. Arrive early for the appointment so you can relax and get ready to talk in detail about the experiences you have been going through. Remember that, your health care provider is there to listen to you, discuss your concerns and find ways to help you. You may be given a questionnaire to fill or it may be an open talk. This will give your health care provider the information that is needed. It will also make him or her to understand and also be able to assess your condition.

The following may help:

- You can either book an appointment to discuss binge eating disorder or you talk about it bring during you regular visits. Carry your notes about the bingeing episodes, the symptoms you have listed and questions you wish to ask the doctor. Keep the purpose of your visit in mind and don't blush it away because it concerns your life and that is why it is important. Stay focused while you are talking and bring up your concerns with your health care provider.

- If you are comfortable with it you may let your doctor know in advance you're your visit is about talking about binge eating disorder so he or she can prepare for it. You may or may not do this before the visit. It depends on what you feel comfortable with. Some people would rather take it up when they are already in the office.

- You may want to take a family member or a friend along with you or you would want to discuss your condition privately.

- Arrive for the appointment before time so you can fill out the forms, go through your notes, and relax. If you arrive on time, you may feel anxious especially if it is your first visit.

- When you get to the office, start the conversation as soon as you can. Talk with your health care provider privately if that is what you want.

- Time may be limited, so start the conversation as soon as you are settled so the doctor can have time to listen and respond to what you say.

- It helps to be specific instead of generalizing. Be specific about your symptoms and describe them in detail.

- Focus on your binge eating condition and make it your top priority when talking with your doctor.

Go for counseling

Counseling helps you to open up about your problems. Binge eating disorders, can be successfully treated with both psychological counseling and nutrition counseling.

- Psychological counseling – is talk therapy. It helps you to come out of hiding to talk with a professional therapist or mental health provider, who understands your problems. The therapist you visit, talk to on phone or in self-help computer-based therapy helps you to recognize or identify thoughts and feelings and which lead you to binge eating. You are taught how you can change them into helpful thoughts, feelings and behaviors (actions).

- Nutrition counseling – is also vital for your recovery. This helps you to have structured meal plans (which you should stick to), healthy eating habits and weight management.

- Medications – such as antidepressants may be prescribed if you are depressed. People who are obese may benefit from medications that control appetite and weight gain.

Treatment and lifestyle changes will definitely have a higher success rate than adopting weight-loss programs. This is due to the fact that you can lose weight and still continue bingeing which adds more weight. You can do get better if your mental condition is treated so you stop bingeing. You could lose weight when you stop bingeing, because you are not overeating as you used to. You will also burn calories when you start healthy foods which have the nutrients the body requires.

Chapter 6:
How Body Dysmorphic Disorder and Binge Eating Disorder Relate. Can you cure one without the other?

Body dysmorphic disorder (BDD) and binge eating disorder (BED) are related and that is why you can't cure one without the other.

Relationship between BDD and BED

They are both mental disorders. It therefore helps to treat these conditional from the mental viewpoint rather than physical. Once the mental problems have been addressed, the physical problems like weight-gain respond positively. However, physical conditions that arise as a result of these disorders should also be treated.

Body dysmorphic disorder and binge eating disorder are body image problems. They involve obsessions and compulsions that you are not able to control until you get therapy. People with BDD worry about their appearance, while those with BED, are worried about their weight, size and shape. Those with BDD fret about an area in their body like the nose while those with BED are concerned with the whole body. They all have distorted thoughts, feelings and behaviors which need to be changed.

People with BDD and BED have an extremely distorted body image. They display a negative body image and low self-esteem. When you have BDD, you are driven by an overwhelming obsession that you are ugly and unattractive. This causes compulsions like looking in the mirror for a long time, picking on the skin and avoiding social interactions. When you have BED you are driven by fear of being obese or overweight. In both cases, you view your body negatively.

Both these conditions involve emotional disturbances such as anxiety, sadness, fear and worry among many others. The people with these disorders have distorted feelings which include moods and physical sensations.

These disorders feed on each other. Individuals who suffer from BDD have eating disorders mainly binge eating disorder. When you have a problem with your body image, you tend to be in low moods and have low self-esteem. You may develop stress or depression. This can cause you to seek comfort in foods. As a result of finding relief in food, you can find yourself doing this over and over again which may result in binge eating.

The diagnosis of both these conditions is intertwined in many ways. It involves uncovering problems that would have caused these problems. These could be genetic predisposition, abuse while one was a child, brain changes and the environment. Since both these problems tend to start either in adolescence or childhood, because of abuse, bullying and other problems, that is why you cannot treat one without treating the other.

It has been observed that, if body dysmorphic disorder remains untreated for a long time, it has a tendency to develop into an eating disorder such as binge eating disorder, bulimia and anorexia. On the other hand, people suffering from eating disorders have a distorted body image which is the same with dysmorphic body disorder. In addition to this, both diseases often share some of the same psychological problems such as stress, anxiety, depression and other problems. These problems ought to be treated so you can live a happy life.

Symptoms

Body dysmorphic disorder and binge eating disorder, are related in many ways. They share similar symptoms which need to be addressed in the treatment plan.

People with BDD and BED obsessively check their appearance in mirrors, they groom excessively by putting on make ups,

Undergoing numerous cosmetic surgery operations without satisfaction

Showing reduced or poor performance at work or school

Utilizing extreme diet and exercise behaviors

They may avoid social situations to hide their problems. Those with BDD hide their flaws whether real or imagined while those with BED hide because their obesity. They stay away from the public eye because of their fear and low self-esteem. They also believe others view them the same way they view themselves and avoid being judged.

They usually compare themselves with others and they feel inadequate or unattractive.

They perform rituals such as touching the skin to smooth it and weighing themselves frequently to see if they have lost weight.

Whether you have BDD or BED, you may seek surgery to correct your flaws or lose weight.

People with BDD may look in the mirror excessively like for 2 hours or more, while those with BED usually eat excessively or they consume large quantities of food within a specific time, like 2 hours.

Those with BDD feel unable to control their rituals and routines while those with BED feel that their eating behavior is out of control. Both have loss of control which should be reinstated by treatment so that they feel confident again. is what makes binge eating disorder different from normal overeating whereby you are able to control the eating.

These people often feel disgusted or upset with their appearance or weight and they may feel depressed, ashamed, or guilty with themselves because of their compulsive habits. They may feel relieved but this is only for a short time. They should seek long-term solutions as we have stated in this book. Putting a lot of make-up and dieting will not solve the problem. Try lifestyle and home remedies recommended in this book or seeking treatment are the only ways you can overcome both disorders.

When you eat large amounts of food in secret or you hide your flaws doesn't help. This is because you end up feeling ashamed or embarrassed. Talk to someone about your problem and open up. You can also join a support group in your area where you will meet other people with similar problems. You will receive advice, and work together towards recovery.

You need to break the vicious cycle. If you are not able to break it on your own, seek help.

There are many complications that can arise as a result of body dysmorphic disorder and binge eating disorder. If you are suffering from body dysmorphic disorder and/or binge eating disorder, you should seek treatment immediately do these conditions can be treated before they become life-threatening.

Using therapy to address body dysmorphic disorder and binge eating disorder can be helpful. In both cases, CBT is very effective. It helps to change any distorted thoughts and perceptions about your body image and it can be combined with medications when necessary to make it more effective. This assures you of long-term recovery so you can have quality of life and a happy meaningful life.

An ultimate goal during treatment for body dysmorphic disorders as well as eating disorders is to help the individual develop a positive self-image and improved self-esteem.

People compulsively overeat because they use food as a way of coping with their negative emotions. Some people who overeat BED and/or BDD but they fail to address their emotional problems. These people end up feeling guilty or ashamed afterward. They may try to stop their negative habits and fail because they are driven by something else other than their compulsions. This is emotions. These people should receive dialectical therapy and interpersonal therapy.

- **Dialectical Behavior Therapy (DBT)** – will help you to learn better skills that help you in your behavior. These are behavioral and coping skills which help you to be able to handle stress and negative emotions. You will learn how to regulate your emotions in a way that you are able to avoid overreactions when you are faced with challenging situations, so you feel in control. Your attitudes towards yourself situations improve by replacing them with healthy ones you no longer feel that your flaws or obesity make you unattractive.

- **Interpersonal psychotherapy** – helps you to improve your relationships with other people so you feel more acceptable whether you have real flaws or obesity. You will find that, as you relate with other people in better ways, your compulsions lessen whether it involves putting on makes-ups to cover your flaws or they involve binge eating, ultimately you will get better and you overcome your condition. You will also be able to resist the urges and you will feel in control of your life.

Factors that may cause BDD and BED

Genetic predisposition: BDD and BED may be as a result of genetic predisposition. These disorders have been observed for a long time and conclusions made that, they run in some families. Both conditions tend to affect those with relatives who have the same condition.

Inherited genes predispose people to these conditions.

Psychological issues: Most people with these disorders have negative issues, about themselves. This may cause the development of these conditions which may be triggered by stress, anxiety, poor body image, low self-esteem and feelings of anger. These should be addressed during treatment.

Age: Anyone can get these disorders but they usually, begin in childhood and adolescence. They occur in childhood because of abuse and criticism while adolescences are too aware of their looks, shape and size. They may also deal with their emotions and low moods in unhealthy ways like over-reacting causing them to develop stress, anxiety and depression. They should get treatment so they can learn skills to handle their emotions and moods in healthy ways rather than over-reacting. Adults should also practice the steps recommended in this book or get treatment to cope with these disorders and ultimately overcome them.

Environment and life experiences: These factors play a major role in the development of body dysmorphic disorder and binge eating disorder. People who suffer from these disorders may have experiences physical abuse, criticism about their body weight, childhood obesity, childhood abuse or stressful and/or traumatic events. These negative experiences about their body or their self-image play a major role in the development of this disorder, because of that environment. People who were teased, bullied or abused when they were children or adolescences may have these disorders.

Other factors that trigger these disorders include emotional conflicts during childhood, low self-esteem in any age even adulthood, parents and other people who criticized their appearance, high expectations from society and peer pressure can lead to development of both BDD and BED. With the right care and treatment both these conditions can be cured.

Brain differences: causes many disorders including body dysmorphic disorder and binge eating disorder among others. That is why antidepressants such as SSRIs are usually prescribed.

Can you cure one without the other?

BED and BDD are related, so treatment should be planned that treat both disorders and other conditions.

What treatment should target

Medical professionals who treat people with either body dysmorphic disorder or binge eating disorder say that, treatment is effective and has long-term benefits when the underlying causes are addressed when this is done, the condition is ultimately eliminated. This may not happen overnight, but when these people take measures to stop unhealthy behaviors and adopt healthy behaviors and attitudes with or without treatment, changes can be noted right away. The doctor and those supporting these people should encourage them to change their attitudes and behaviors either on their own or with help. This helps them to feel in control of their lives and they also feel better about themselves.

In the studies done, therapy showed high long-term success in not only reducing binge eating but in treating body dysmorphic disorder and a wide-range of psychological problems. If you help these people to eliminate unhealthy patterns in their lives, this has a great impact on their body weight and how they view themselves. Some researchers argue that weight-loss should also be addressed and this is done using behavioral weight-loss programs, which are usually less expensive and effective within a short time especially if they are supervised.

Many people who use behavioral weight-loss programs say that it helps to eliminate obesity especially when combined with therapy.

Treatment for BDD and BED is more effective when people don't have other medical conditions. This means that the conditions can be addressed without other serious psychological problems. That is why you should take steps to overcome binge eating disorder and body dysmorphic disorder as early as possible before other complication start developing. If someone has more long-term, psychological or physical difficulties then treatment should address all these problems. Some patients, especially those with depression need specialized treatment.

Support

There are many groups, which include formal and formal ones. Some are supervised by a therapist while others are not.

- Individualized psychological therapy – is a one-on-one therapy for individuals such as CBT. Therapy takes place between the therapist and patient.

- Group therapy – is therapy given to a group facing the same challenges. It is led by a trained therapist or volunteer.

Anything that affects the group members may be discussed whether it is about binge eating or healthy eating. Members discuss about their experiences while giving and receiving advice as they support one other.

- Self-help books – read alone or with a support group and share ideas.

- Online courses – can be taken alone or as part of a support group

- Supervised self-help programs – guided by a professional by having regular contacts usually on phone.

Avoid the Risk Factors

The best way to overcome BDD and BED is to avoid the risk factors which you can, as much as possible. Some factors have a tendency to increase the risk of developing or even worsening these conditions or they may trigger them.

- You may not choose where and in which family you will be corn but knowing that you have biological relatives with body dysmorphic disorder and binge eating disorders helps you to take preventative measures. This could be eating healthy foods, watching warning signs or seeking help early enough before these conditions worsen. You can adopt the steps we have recommended by making lifestyle changes.

- You may not have been able to prevent the negative life experiences that you have gone through like childhood abuse, criticism and bullying, but you have the power to stop them destroying your life. Talk to someone. Confront your past and address it. Yes it happened and the damage was done but you can pick the pieces of what was left and mend them together.

- You can change your personality traits which make you have low self-esteem and feel unacceptable.

- The society has its own expectations that may lead you to view beauty and attractiveness differently. Just know that you are unique and there is no one like you in this whole world.

- Having anxiety disorder or depression should not stop you from being whom you want to be.

Complications

There are many complications that are caused by these disorders. These complications should be addressed otherwise they can worsen the medical conditions you have. If they are not treated they can complicate the treatments you may be receiving.

- Stress and depression require specialized treatment but they can be treated successful.

- High blood pressure can develop due to obesity, stress and other causes. If you have high blood pressure you need to have the condition managed. Talk to your doctor about ways to prevent this condition. Avoid the problem by taking life easily and dealing with stress in healthy ways as we have explained. Avoid any triggers that make you to over-react when faced with challenging situations.

- High cholesterol levels may be caused by eating unhealthy foods which are loaded with unhealthy fats causing your body to store "bad" cholesterol in the body. However, you should know that, not all cholesterol is bad; there is "good" cholesterol that the body requires to function properly.

- Type 2 diabetes may be caused by high blood sugar in the body, and the inability of the body systems, to get rid of it. When you consume foods rich in sugar especially simple carbohydrates i.e. junk foods and those loaded with refined sugar like packaged products, the blood sugar rises suddenly. This requires more insulin to be produced in the body to get rid of the excess blood sugar. The sudden rise and fall of blood sugar in the body causes problems. The body systems also concentrate on getting rid of the sugar in the blood instead of eliminating toxins and performing other functions in the body which causes more problems. That is why you should consume healthy foods all the time.

- Cardiovascular diseases, stroke and coronary heart disease may be caused by obesity. This may be due to a number of factors like deposits of the bad cholesterol in the blood vessels and other factors.

- Osteoarthritis, joint and muscle pain may be present in cases where people gain weight and become obese.

- Gall bladder disease and gastrointestinal problems are other conditions that may be found in people with obesity.

People with BDD and BED may have difficulty attending work or school. They like avoiding the public because of their "imperfections". This doesn't make things better for them. Coming out in the open may be possible after therapy or when they receive encouragement from family or friends as well as their support groups. Having social phobia and isolation happens because they believe other people view them the same way they view themselves. Therapy exposes them to these situations to help them cope. They also learn skills to help them develop close and stable relationships with family or friends which make them confident and able to go out and face the world.

Prevention

Prevention is better than curing an already existing problem. That is why you should find ways to prevent body dysmorphic disorder and binge eating disorder. As soon as you notice the symptoms, start treatment right away. But the best way to prevent these disorders altogether is to follow the steps and tips we have recommended throughout this book. Any steps taken in the right direction will deter the development of these disorders.

If you are prone to these disorders, you should adopt healthy attitudes and behaviors as taught in cognitive behavioral therapy and other types of therapies explained in this book. Try as much as possible to view yourself realistically. Many people have flaws and other things that make them different but they don't become obsessed with their body image. No one way created perfect even those people you regard as your role models. They are only who they are because they are able to deal with their problems positively. Don't look at yourself negatively, be positive. This will help to prevent the development and triggering of BDD and BED.

If you already have these disorders, do what is recommended in this book to prevent these conditions worsening and leading to more complications. Identify the root cause of your problem and confront it. You may have been bullies as a child or teens and you didn't deal with it at that time. It is never too late. The right time is now you realize that, something went wrong. Talk to someone and open up about the problem. A problem shared is a problem half-solved. You may have been criticized in the past. Let me encourage you, you can rise above your problem and live a meaningful life. Listen to motivational speakers on TV, audio tapes or read their books. You will be surprised to learn that, there are many people who are out there who had similar problems but they didn't allow their problems to hold them back. They have moved to great heights despite their challenges.

Chapter 7:
How Both Can be Signs of Personality Disorders

Best therapies and methods to deal with these personality disorders

If you have binge eating disorder and body dysmorphic disorder there is hope for you. Bothe these conditions can be signs of personality disorders. These are mental disorders which cause people to have distorted views about themselves and may behave in ways that differ from the average person. Binge eating disorder causes people to have negative thoughts, feelings, moods and behaviors just like people with BDD. These people may have problems with their personalities and how they relate with other people.

- Odd behavior – someone with binge eating behavior usually eats large amounts of food and continues eating even when full. People with BDD look at themselves in the mirror for hours or pick on their skin and fret too much about their physical appearance. These and other habits are odd behaviors.

- Stress and depression – are common in people with both BED and BDD. The best treatment approach is to have these underlying problems addressed.

- Becoming overwhelmed by anxiety, anger, distress, and worthlessness – is common in people with either BED or BDD or both. These people may have anxiety disorders, express themselves with anger outbursts and feel distresses. They may feel worthless and attach little or no value to themselves because of their overeating in binge eating disorder or their appearance in body dysmorphic disorder. In the most extreme cases, they may have suicidal thoughts or commit suicide. Both conditions are complex and so treatment and prevention should be addressed. Fortunately, anyone can get better if what is recommended in this book is applied.

- Avoiding social interactions and feeling emotionally disconnected – many people with binge eating disorder eat in secret and they hide their problem. This also happens with people who have dysmorphic disorder. They avoid social interactions and going out in public because of their appearance. People with either of these disorders have a negative self-image about themselves. Luckily we have listen they can take to overcome these problems.

- Difficulty with relationships, especially maintaining close and stable relationships with spouse, children, work colleagues, and professional care workers. This is true about both these disorders. Interpersonal therapy can help you to cultivate healthy relationships with other people.

- Losing contact with the reality – people with personality disorders lose contact with reality. They have distorted beliefs which should be challenged and CBT helps them do this and face life realistically.

- Difficulty coping with negative feelings which may lead to self-harm – these disorders become more complicated when someone has depression and other medical conditions. Treatment should be sought for these medical conditions.

- Abusing drugs or alcohol, or taking medication drug overdoses – some people feel hopeless because of their condition and start substance abuse. This only complicates the problem. You can start recovery once you start withdrawing from drugs or alcohol and other things that trigger the symptoms. Ask your doctor where you can find support groups in your areas. Remember, your family and friends love you and you should reach out to them for support.

- Threatening others – is rare although it can happen when someone has depression.

Causes of Personality Disorders

There are several causes of personality disorders

- Genetic predispositions – can be the cause of binge eating or body dysmorphic disorder.

- Life experiences such as trauma or abuse – can contribute to the development and trigger of these conditions.

- Child abuse whether physical, emotional or verbal, and neglect – may be the underlying problem that makes you have a problem with your self-image.

You can recover with time and in most cases, support is all that you need. These disorders improve when you receive psychotherapy while at times, therapy is combined with medications to be effective.

Best therapies and methods to deal with these personality disorders

There are many therapies and methods available for treating personality disorders such as body dysmorphic disorder and binge eating disorder among others. Treatment may include individualized therapy, family therapy or group therapy as well as computerized therapy among others as we shall see in this chapter. Medications which are prescribed by a qualified doctor may be helpful in alleviating symptoms of personality disorders which include anxiety and depression as we have seen in earlier chapters.

Treatment of these personality disorders

1. Psychological Therapies

- Psychotherapy

- CBT

- Interpersonal Therapy

- Psychodynamic or Reflective Psychotherapy

2. Therapeutic Communities

3. Medications

Psychological Therapies

All psychological therapies should be conducted by trained therapists because they deal with sensitive conditions that are considered high-risk. The aim of psychological therapies is to help the patients to regulate their thoughts, emotions and behaviors. The therapist can focus on either your negative or dysfunctional thought patterns, guide you towards self-reflection and make you understand how your mind works so you can influence it positively. Group therapies enhance understanding of social relationships.

Psychological therapies are effective in treating personality disorders especially body dysmorphic disorder and binge eating disorder. However, the therapist must be trained and have the right experience to handle these high-risk conditions which, if not well handled may lead to destructive behaviors such as self-harm. That is why the patient should be handled carefully. The therapist you choose should have the right training and experience of working with personality disorders with significant success. When choosing a trained professional, ask for referrals from family and friends or ask your family doctor for recommendations.

Psychotherapy

Psychotherapy is treatment involves the patient and a trained therapist having a discussion about the patient's thoughts, emotions and behaviors ether on their own or with family or in group sessions. The psychotherapist will listen and discuss important issues that affect your life with you or your family and work with you to change your thoughts, attitudes and behaviors. This includes practicable strategies that will help to resolve the problems you are having so that you can overcome them and live a meaningful life.

Psychotherapy will focus on helping you to uncover unconscious conflicts that have contributed to your disorder some of which may have started in childhood or adolescence. This will help you to discover the cause of your symptoms because it is only then that you can be able to find lasting solutions. Psychotherapy also helps you to change the negative or inappropriate behavior patterns like overeating and purging or having a poor body image and hiding from other people because of your perceived appearance that interfere with your everyday living.

In psychotherapy, you also realize that your behavior affects other people as well. This may be your parents, spouse or children, they may be your friends or work colleagues or the public. This helps you to cultivate close and stable relationships with those you love and care about as well as people in general whether you meet them on the street, on the internet or elsewhere. You are able to recognize the effect your behavior has on others so that you focus on changing your attitudes and behavior to be more acceptable.

Cognitive behavioral therapy

CBT is based on the theory that your thoughts, feelings and behavior are inter-related and each affects the other. This means that, the way you think about an event or situation affects how you act. On the other hand, your actions affect how you think and feel. It is necessary to change your thinking (cognition) and behave (behavior).

CBT is an effective therapy that helps you to manage your problems by changing the way you think and behave. You'll need to agree with your therapist on your therapy goals, so you can work towards the same goals. You will also need to plan the sessions in terms of the number of sessions you need to attend and the durations whether you will receive therapy as an individual, with your family or as a group. An important part of CBT is graded exposure and response prevention (ERP). This is performed in supervised therapy where the therapist guides you to face normal situations like where the food you cave is available if you are a binge eater or situations which you would normally fret over your appearance if you have body dysmorphic disorder. You are exposed to the problem and you try and control your response. ERP helps you to gradually cope with these situations in better ways over time.

CBT is a type of psychotherapy which recognizes that thoughts, feelings and behaviors are interrelated. Thoughts affect feelings which influence actions or behaviors. You can change the way you feel and behave by the way you think which helps you to cope with your problems. CBT involves individual counseling or family and/or group therapy. It focuses on changing your thinking (cognitive therapy) and your behavior (behavioral therapy) if you have body dysmorphic disorder or other mental illnesses.

The aim of cognitive behavioral therapy is to help you to learn as much as possible about your disorder, your thoughts, feelings moods and behavior. It also shows you how to use what you have learnt to stop automatic negative thoughts so you can be positive and realistic about how you see yourself and others. CBT helps you to learn healthy ways to influence your behavior, by controlling your eating habits, checking yourself in the mirror or avoiding it and such behaviors. This helps you to handle the compulsive and obsessive routines or rituals in better ways by gaining control of your life. It also teaches you how to socialize with other people and other helpful behaviors.

You and your therapist will need to discuss about the type of therapy that is appropriate for you.

Psychodynamic or Reflective Psychotherapy

Psychodynamic psychotherapy is based on the fact that many of the problems that cause adult patterns of behavior stem back from early childhood. The patient may have gone through negative childhood experiences which caused distorted thinking and beliefs which formed behavioral patterns. As long as one was a child, these behaviors were understood in that context but when the person became an adult and continued to behave the same way then they are considered as personality disorders.

The main goal of reflective psychotherapy is to explore in depth what these distorted behaviors are, how they arose, and how they can be resolved effectively. You will work with your therapist to find practical ways to overcome these distortions and ensure that they don't influence your thoughts and behavior. You can have individualized or group psychodynamic therapy or a combination of both. This may be helpful in overcoming not only body dysmorphic disorder and binge eating disorder but other personality disorders as well.

Interpersonal therapy

Interpersonal therapy (IPT) is shown to be an effective type of therapy in many mental disorders. Your relationship with other people is important. The way the people around you view and treat you and the way you view and treat them, is crucial to your well-being. We are social animals and we have needs to love and belong. If you feel isolated or you avoid social interactions because of your problems like having problems with your appearance, then your relationships suffer and this affects your mental health whether you know it or not.

Interpersonal therapy is based on the fact that, your relationships with other people and the world at large have a great effect on your mental health. This is why when you have problems interacting with other people it may lead you to have feelings of anxiety, low self-esteem, self-doubt and lack of confidence. When you attend therapy sessions, your therapist will discuss about your interpersonal relationships to explore any negative experiences and any issues you may be having with other people in order to work with you to resolve the problems. This will improve your relationships with others and the way you view and interpret the world in general.

Therapeutic Communities

Therapeutic communities (TCs) are a type of group therapy or community therapy as the name suggests. It is a very intensive form of therapy which requires commitment on the part of the patient for it to become effective. The group therapy explores in depth the patient's experience of the personality disorder whether it is binge eating disorder, dysmorphic disorder and other conditions to find the root cause of the problem in order to resolve it. Everything is explored in depth. TCs are known to be effective especially in the treatment of mild to moderate personality disorders.

Medications

SSRIs antidepressants are the most commonly used medications used to treat body dysmorphic disorder and binge eating disorder. Other medications include psychiatric medications used for treating depression. These medications are shown to be effective especially the selective serotonin reuptake inhibitors (SSRIs) antidepressants prescribed for BDD and BED. They are known to be safer and have fewer side effects than other medications and that is why they are highly recommended. SSRIs work by increasing the serotonin levels, in the brain lifting the patient's moods and emotions therefore suppressing some of the symptoms of these disorders.

SSRIs are known to be more effective than other antidepressants. They stabilize the bran so that you are able to control your obsessions and compulsions whether in binge eating episodes or in behavioral dysmorphic disorder. The dosage depends on the individual, the severity of the problem and the circumstances. The doctor may start you on lower dosages increasing the dose gradually, as you tolerate the medications. Always take your medications without fail and don't skip taking them so you can get better and improve with time. Sticking to your treatment plan also prevents relapses. You should only withdraw from medications when your doctor recommends it and this is done gradually to minimize any possibility of adverse withdrawal symptoms.

CBT Therapy for binge eating and body dysmorphic therapy

Both binge eating disorder and body dysmorphic disorder can be treated with the types of therapy described in this chapter and other parts of this book. Therapy has shown significant success and recovery is possible. The forms of therapy teach you how to overcome any compulsions and obsessions you may have and how to overcome your problems whether you have BED or BDD or both. You learn how to replace unhealthy habits with healthy ones.

The most commonly used therapy is CBT and that is why we have decided to cover it in detail in this part of the book.

What is Cognitive Behavioral Therapy?

Cognitive behavioral therapy (CBT) is a type of psychotherapy or talking therapy that is used to treat binge eating disorder and body dysmorphic disorder as well as other mental disorders and addictions. Although CBT was originally developed for treating anxiety and depression, it is used today to treat a wide-range of mental illnesses and physical health problems.

CBT is based on the theory that your thoughts, feelings and behaviors affect each other. When you have negative thoughts and feelings they automatically lead you to have negative behaviors or actions. When you have negative behaviors, they make you feel bad and lead you to have negative thoughts and feelings. This forms negative patterns which keep going on and on and unless you stop them, you may be trapped in a vicious cycle. Take for example; if you are a binge eater, you eat excessively, then you diet or skip meals to compensate for the excess food you have eaten. This causes you to crave for more food which leads to more over-eating. Luckily, CBT aims to help you break this vicious cycle. It teaches you how to change the negative patterns of behavior to improve the way you feel. This improves your thinking as well.

CBT is most commonly used to treat anxiety and depression, but it is useful in the treatment of all mental disorders and addictions. CBT will help you deal with your problems in a more positive way so you can cope with them and to ultimately overcome them completely. You feel in control again.

The therapist will focus his or her attention on examining the relationship between your thoughts, feelings and behaviors, then, explore the patterns of thinking that lead you to unhealthy feelings and behaviors. You should know that, thoughts and feelings are the main contributory factors to your behaviors or actions. Therapists try to find out the root cause of the problem by examining your belief systems which could be distorted or unrealistic. Your belief system is powerful in directing thoughts either positively or negatively. If you are helped to modify your patterns of thinking, it should in turn improve your coping mechanisms and overcome your problems.

Benefits derived from CBT

- CBT is a highly structured treatment that is available in many different forms including self-help books, face-to face one-on-one sessions, family and group therapy and computerized cognitive behavioral therapy.

- Cognitive behavioral therapy is known to be more effective than medications in treating body dysmorphic disorder, binge eating disorders, mood disorders and addictions such as stress, anxiety, depression and phobias. However, patients need to participate and be committed to the therapy in order to practice the skills learnt.

- Therapy can be done alone or combined with medications to enhance their effectiveness. This therapy may be helpful where medications have failed to be effective.

- CBT deals with current problems and not past problems although they are taken into consideration, and that is why it is effective, within a short period of time unlike other talking therapies.

- The skills learnt are helpful, practical and effective. You should practice them daily to prevent relapses. Let them become part of your life so you can overcome these mental disorders. Maintain them in your whole life an you will find life meaningful.

- Use CBT to prevent any mental and physical problems from recurring.

When you can use cognitive behavioral therapy

CBT is an effective way of treating all types of mental disorders and addictions among other health conditions. The principles which are stated in this book can be used in any type of mental disorder, relationship problems, physical problems, drug or alcohol addictions and other mental illnesses. There are some severe conditions like depression which require a combination of CBT and medications.

How CBT works

You already have some knowledge about CBT from what you have read earlier in this book. Whether you are working on binge eating disorder, body dysmorphic disorder or other problems, your therapist will break down cognitive behavioral therapy into 5 main areas:

- Situations

- Thoughts

- Physical feelings

- Emotions

- Actions or behavior

Cognitive behavioral therapy is usually based on the above five main areas. These factors are interconnected and they therefore affect each other. You need to understand them so you can be able to use them to overcome your problems. A situation can arise at any time like when you see food. This makes you interpret or attach some meaning to the food, let us say "good food" which leads to thoughts. You may think "I am hungry" even when you are not. These hunger thoughts you have about food affect your physical feelings (you start feeling hungry or having cravings) and emotions (you start feeling anxious) which lead to your behavior or actions (over-eating).

If your thoughts about your body image and situations are negative then your feelings and actions will be affected negatively. This means that if you view yourself as overweight because of what you have done (over-eating) you start feeling ashamed, disgusted and guilty. These feelings lead you to diet or skip meals so you can lose weight. This causes cravings and you even eat in secret. One thing leads to another and a pattern is formed.

How CBT can help you

CBT will help you to be in control of your life by changing what you think (you are hungry) which changes what you do (over-eating), which changes how you feel (ashamed, disgusted and guilty). It changes your negative thoughts to positive thoughts which lead to positive actions helping you get better whether you have BED, BDD or other conditions. CBT aims at helping you to break down the things that make you to have those negative thoughts and emotions, so, you can stop feeling negatively about yourself, other people and situations. It also helps you to change your negative attitudes to positive ones. It helps you to deal with the problems you may be having and make them more manageable. It is true that, you cannot change some situations like if you had abuse, criticisms and bullying, but, you can change the way you feel about them. A trained therapist will help you to tackle these problems by changing your thoughts to improve the way you feel and behave which makes you get better. After some time, you will be able to do this on your own without the help of a therapist.

CBT sessions

Cognitive behavioral therapy can be individualized therapy between a trained therapist and yourself in one-on-one sessions or family sessions whether a family members like your mother, father, sibling, child or spouse can accompany you for therapy or it can be group therapy of people with similar problems. Others can help you to manage the problem if you work together. Mental problems affect the whole family so it is important to get help as a family in family therapy. The family members can provide you with support which you need.

They can notice warning signs which trigger the problem and help you to take the necessary measure. Family therapy also makes you accountable to your loved and this helps you to remain focused on your therapy goals. Therapy can be given to groups of people who have similar problems.

You can therefore get therapy as an individual, as a family or as a group. The sessions may last 30 to 60 minutes which depends on the severity of the problem. Group sessions can take 2 ½ hours or longer so everyone can have a chance to participate. Exposure therapy sessions take longer to ensure that your symptoms whether they involve fear or anxiety, are significantly reduced during these sessions. The therapist can be a healthcare professional who is trained in CBT such as a psychologist, a psychiatrist or a general physician or a psychiatric nurse.

The first CBT session

The first session starts by the therapist talking with you and explaining what CBT which is followed by an initial assessment of your mental disorder. The CBT therapist will ask you questions about your life and the symptoms you have been experiencing. This is to help him or her to determine whether CBT is the appropriate therapy for you or you require other types of therapy. The therapist will also want to know if you are comfortable with CBT.

The therapist will base the questions on:

- Your life and background. If you have had childhood abuse, criticism and bullying which could have caused the mental disorders.

- Your belief systems i.e. childhood upbringing, family beliefs and values, past experiences. These could be distorted in which case the therapist will ask you to challenge your belief system to be realistic.

- Whether you are stressed, anxious or depressed which could trigger these mental disorders or worsen them.

- Symptoms which you have due to your condition. It helps to list them down before your visit.

- Whether your condition interferes with your family, school, work and your social life.

- Events and situations that may be related to your condition.

- Treatments you have received and their effectiveness

- Your therapy goals or what you intend to achieve with CBT therapy

After answering these questions and CBT seems to be the appropriate kind of treatment for you, the therapist will explain to you what to expect from treatment and make plans when you can attend face-to-face therapy sessions. If CBT is recommended, you will have one session each week or each fortnight up to 5-20 sessions depending on your condition. Some therapists recommend 5-20 sessions while others recommend 6-18 sessions but you can always have a booster when you need further therapy. Each session will last for 30-60 minutes usually and you will have "breaks" of 1-3 weeks between sessions when you can do your "homework" assignments which should be completed before the commencement of the next session.

The assignment may be a simple one like facing your fears for someone with phobia, attending a social event for someone who is depressed or if you are anxious you may be asked by the therapist to talk to a stranger or anything else which you will be able to do. Completing the assignment shows how dedicated you are to the treatment and if you have the desire to change and achieve the goals you have set. After the completion of your assignment and how successful you were in handling it, the therapist will be able to plan the next session and the activities to give you. During "breaks" it may help to have real time counseling with your therapist through computer links or over the phone.

If this type of therapy is not appropriate for you or you don't feel comfortable with it, you will be given recommendations of alternative therapies and other treatments.

Follow-up sessions

Immediately after the assessment sessions, your therapist will start working with you as an individual or as a group to break down your problems into situations, thoughts, emotions, physical feelings and actions as we have seen earlier. You may be asked to write down on a diary about your thoughts and behaviors to see the patterns they form. You and your therapist will work together to analyze your thoughts, feelings and behaviors (actions) to see if they are unrealistic, irrational or unhelpful thoughts.

Together you will check and see how your thoughts, feelings and behaviors are interconnected and how they affect each other, how they affect you and others around you, such as family and colleagues. Your therapist will help you to change your unhelpful thoughts and behaviors and replace them with alternative thoughts which are helpful.

How to stop the negative cycle

We all respond to situations in ways that are either helpful or unhelpful. Research studies have shown that, the way people interpret a situation or the meaning they give to it, is what causes feelings and emotions. If something bad happens to you at a given time, you may feel angry, sad, lonely, hopeless, guilty or depressed. The way you respond to certain situations, depends on whether you have positive or negative thoughts about those situations. If these negative feelings and emotions are not dealt with in a positive way, they may be followed by negative actions like withdrawal from people, violence, self-hate, addictions and other problems.

When you are trapped is such negative thoughts, your actions make you feel even worse and this causes worse actions and the whole scenario repeats itself. But should you allow this to go on and on? No. If we allow this to go on, we allow things to go out of control as we go on a downward spiral. Even when you don't believe it, just know that you have power over it. You can stop the downward spiral and turn it around to your benefit.

We say that, most of what we go through in life is not about what happens to us, but how we react to what happens. There are many situations that are beyond our control like natural calamities such as earthquakes, floods, tsunamis and other weather conditions so we have enough worries to care about. Yet, even those situations which are within our control don't always go the way we want. We are left feeling guilty, scared, anxious, depressed, tired and all that. At times people take drugs and alcohol to escape from reality and before they know it they have become addicts. Some puff a cigarette and before they know it, they are hooked. Think of situations which you have experienced which have made you to feel the way you do and write them down.

What to expect during CBT sessions

Effective cognitive behavioral therapy depends on how successful the healthcare provider and the patient interact. CBT is unlike other forms of psychotherapy because the patient is very involved. The homework assignment should start with simple things before moving to more difficult assignments. You should work at easier assignment first, so you can feel comfortable with the process. You should also feel free to talk to the therapist who should be willing to listen and be flexible enough to work with you in different situations. The changes you have made will be measured to know the effectiveness of the therapy. After working out changes to thoughts and behavior, your therapist will ask you to practice the changes you have learnt in your daily life.

After a few sessions or during self-help therapy you should challenge upsetting thoughts and replace them with alternative thoughts which are helpful. Keep practicing until you can recognize when you are about to do something that is irrational which will ultimately make you feel bad. Correct this potential behavior by doing something helpful and this will make you feel better. This will motivate you even more to change your thoughts and actions and you will feel better and better. You will do more "homework" assignments between CBT sessions moving to more and more difficult scenarios. During each session, you will need to discuss with your therapist about the changes you have made and how it felt. Your therapist will make suggestions to help you with the process.

Exposure therapy can be difficult at first when you start confronting your fears and anxieties. If you fear spiders, you can start by looking at their pictures. Later, you can watch them in enclosed places until you cope with that. Your therapist will not in any way ask you to do things that you don't want to do. You will work at the pace that you are comfortable with. During the CBT sessions whether you are working as an individual or as a group, your therapist will encourage and reassure you, but will also check to see that you are quite comfortable with the treatment progress.

One of the benefits of CBT is that, after you have completed your course, you will be able to continue to apply the skills and the principles that you have learnt in your daily life. When you do this regularly, you will prevent a relapse and ensure that the symptoms do not return. The ultimate aim of CBT is to train you to apply the skills that you have learnt during the treatment sessions to your daily life all your life. This should help you to manage your mood disorders and addictions and stop them from controlling your life and having a negative impact on you and others currently and into the future after you have completed treatment.

How CBT helps you

CBT is different from other types of psychotherapy, in that, the therapist and you as the patient actively work together on one-on-one sessions or with your family members or groups members, to help you to recover. However, for CBT to be effective and have long-lasting effects, the patient has to be actively involved. There is no way that this kind of therapy can work without you playing your role. It is therefore a very interactive type of treatment where you are involved in doing some activities which are analyzed before new activities are developed. You may be involved in group activities but you should also do the assignments you are given.

This therapy is based on the concept that states that, the patient's thoughts, feelings and actions are all interconnected in a way. Negative thoughts and feelings trap patients into a vicious cycle which they find hard to break out of. The therapist aims at helping patients to break-up this cycle and become free from being controlled by moods, emotions and addictions. If you are suffering from any mental disorder or addictions, the therapist will help you to break the problem down into smaller parts which can be dealt with each at a time so that, you are able to change the negative patterns in your life, to improve your feelings, thoughts and behaviors.

In any situation, CBT helps you to be in control by changing what you think which changes what you do, which changes how you feel. It can change negative thoughts to positive thoughts which lead to positive actions helping you feel better. CBT aims at helping you to break down those things that make you have negative thoughts and emotions so you can stop feeling the way you do. It helps you to deal with the problems you have making them more manageable. It is true that, you cannot change some situations but you can change the way you feel about them. Self-help book or professional therapy with a trained therapist helps you to tackle the problems changing your negative thoughts to improve the way you feel. With time, you are able to achieve this on your own without the help of a therapist.

CBT concentrates on your present problems unlike other therapies which try to resolve past problems. By untangling the current problems, you get better much faster than when you try to untangle past problems. This doesn't mean your past is ignored. No. The past is part of your life. By helping you recover from your current conditions somehow, you also solve past problems by changing your attitudes and how you view your past.

Cognitive Behavioral Therapy Sessions

Cognitive behavioral therapy can be provided by a trained therapist in one-on-one sessions between the patient and the therapist. Family members like your mother, father, sibling or spouse can accompany you so they can help you to manage the problem. Furthermore, problems affect the whole family so it is important to get help as a family. It also makes you accountable to them which in a way keep you focused on your goals whether it is to improve your moods or break a bad habit.

Therapy can be given to groups of people who are in similar situations.

If you have CBT you can therefore get therapy as an individual, as a family or as a group. The therapist will give you sessions which last 30-60 minutes depending on the severity of the problem although group sessions can take 2 ½ hours each or longer. Exposure therapy sessions usually take much longer to ensure that your anxiety has significantly reduced during each session.

Therapy can take place in the therapist's clinic, in your home if you have obsessive compulsive disorder or agoraphobia of specific things at home such as the stairs, pets or the darkness, or you can have it outside if you have phobias or fears of things that are outside like swimming pools, spiders and animals. Your therapist can be a healthcare professional who has been specifically trained in CBT such as a psychologist, a psychiatrist or a General Physician or it can be a psychiatric nurse.

What to expect in the first CBT session

Therapy sessions start with the therapist having and initial assessment of your condition whether it is body dysmorphic disorder or binge eating disorder or both. In the first few sessions, the CBT therapist talks with you and asks you or your family member who has accompanied you several questions. You may also be asked to complete a questionnaire and other forms which help to determine whether cognitive behavioral therapy is the most appropriate therapy for you or other therapies should be adopted or combined with CBT. The meaning of CBT is explained to you and you will be asked if you will be comfortable with this type of therapy.

The therapist will ask you questions which may be based on:

- Your life and background, the environment you live in and your belief system. These include your childhood upbringing, family beliefs and values as well as your past experiences.

- If you have stress, anxiety and depressions.

- Whether you have been receiving treatment and which ones.

- The symptoms you experience and if you have other medical conditions.

- If your body dysmorphic disorder and/or binge eating disorder, interfere with your family, school, work and social life.

- The events and situations which may be related to your condition to determine the root cause of the problem.

- If the treatments have been effective.

- Your therapy goals and what you intend to achieve with CBT therapy.

When you answer these questions you will be given time to ask questions about your concerns. It helps to write what you need to know on a piece of paper or notebook before you go for the therapy session. If it is found that CBT is the right treatment for you, the therapist will explain to you what you should expect from therapy. You will discuss treatment plan i.e. how many sessions are necessary, how long each therapy will take, if face-to-face therapy, family therapy or group therapy is the most appropriate or a combinations of therapies is better for you. An appointment is booked for your next therapy session. You will be told when you can attend your next face-to-face therapy sessions or others.

If CBT is recommended, you will have one therapy session every week or every fortnight ranging from 5 to 20 sessions which depend on the severity of your condition. If you require more therapy sessions, your therapist will let you know. Most therapy sessions last for 30-60 minutes or more but you will be given breaks of 1-3 weeks between the sessions when you can do your assignments at home. These may include going out with a family member or friend, going to social interactions and other homework.

When you come for the next therapy session, your therapist will check the homework and discuss with you what you did and what challenges you faced. That is Completing the assignment shows how dedicated you are to the treatment and if you have the desire to change and achieve the goals you have set. After the completion of your assignment and how successful you were in handling it, the therapist will be able to plan the next session and the activities to give you. During "breaks" it may help to have real time counseling with your therapist through computer links or over the phone.

If this type of therapy is not appropriate for you or you don't feel comfortable receiving it, the therapist may recommend alternative therapies and treatments.

Follow-up sessions

Immediately after the assessment sessions, your therapist will start working with you as an individual or as a group to break down your problems into situations, thoughts, emotions, physical feelings and actions as we have seen earlier. You may be asked to write down on a diary about your thoughts and behaviors to see the patterns they form. You and your therapist will work together to analyze your thoughts, feelings and behaviors (actions) to see if they are unrealistic, irrational or unhelpful thoughts. Together you will check and see how your thoughts, feelings and behaviors are interconnected and how they affect each other, how they affect you and others around you, such as family and colleagues. Your therapist will help you to change your unhelpful thoughts and behaviors and replace them with alternative thoughts which are helpful.

How you can apply CBT in your life

Cognitive behavioral therapy (CBT) is used to treat mental disorders which may also cause physical problems. When the disorders are treated, whether in therapy sessions or using computer-based cognitive behavioral therapy (CCBT), physical problems also disappear. However, you need to participate and have the desire to overcome your problems. In addition to therapy, you will also benefit by making lifestyle changes which we have recommended.

You can apply self-help CBT in your life by following these steps:

- Identify your negative thoughts, feelings (physical sensations and moods) and behaviors

- Understand the links between thoughts, feelings and behaviors

- Challenge your thoughts and beliefs

- Make changes to your thoughts and behaviors

CBT is a combination of psychotherapy and behavioral therapy and that is why it is popular. Psychotherapy as the name indicates deals with your mind while behavioral therapy deals with your behavior. Psychotherapy concentrates on changing your distorted beliefs and the importance you attach to certain things like binge eating and your appearance. It helps you to challenge these beliefs which are unrealistic. Take for example, you may believe that you cannot control your eating or you are ugly and unattractive. This is not true. Therapy exposes you to real situations and helps you deal with them realistically. It changes what you belief and you become realistic.

Behavioral therapy deals with your behavior which is influenced by your thoughts and feelings. If you think you are ugly, you hide from people. Therapy helps you to correct your negative actions. CBT has gained popularity among therapists and patients because of its ability to treat mental disorders successfully. It is practiced by general practitioners, psychologists, psychiatrists, social workers, nurses who have the necessary training in CBT.

Computerized cognitive behavioral therapy (CCBT)

Computerized cognitive behavioral therapy (CCBT) is also known as internet-delivered cognitive behavioral therapy (ICBT). The advancement in technology and availability of the internet has encouraged the development of interactive software programs which you can use without the help of a therapist. There are computer packages that have proved effective in the treatment of mild to moderate disorders although it is better to take them with support. If you don't have support, you may be tempted to drift back to your old ways because you have no one you are accountable to. You can start CCBT alone if you are determined. If you falter, you can keep trying or seek support.

Computerized cognitive behavioral therapy (CCBT) is preferred by some people who don't want to open up about their problems. They prefer it instead of going for face-to-face sessions with a therapist or in group sessions. This is because CCBT is private and cost-effective. Computerized cognitive behavioral therapy (CCBT) makes it easier for you to access therapies and avoid the high costs of face-to-face therapy. It is also popular where it is hard to get affordable professional therapists.

Reading self-help books and CCBT are effective ways to treat mild to moderate mental disorders and they are often cheaper than face-to-face therapy. In severe cases it is advisable to seek professional help so intensive therapy can be given or combined with medications. Seeking professional help is also necessary because you may have other medical conditions which worsen symptoms.

Some people prefer to read CBT self-help books or use computerized cognitive behavioral therapy (CCBT) instead of talking to a therapist about their problems. However, it is good to have occasional face-to-face sessions with your therapist or talk over the phone so the professional therapist can guide you through the recovery process as well as monitor your progress.

How you can apply CBT in your life

Cognitive behavioral therapy (CBT) is used to treat mental disorders which may also cause physical problems. When the disorders are treated, whether in therapy sessions or using computer-based cognitive behavioral therapy (CCBT), physical problems also disappear. However, you need to participate and have the desire to overcome your problems. In addition to therapy, you will also benefit by making lifestyle changes which we have recommended.

You can apply self-help CBT in your life by following these steps:

- Identify your negative thoughts, feelings (physical sensations and moods) and behaviors

- Understand the links between thoughts, feelings and behaviors

- Challenge your thoughts and beliefs

- Make changes to your thoughts and behaviors

CBT is a combination of psychotherapy and behavioral therapy and that is why it is popular. Psychotherapy as the name indicates deals with your mind while behavioral therapy deals with your behavior. Psychotherapy concentrates on changing your distorted beliefs and the importance you attach to certain things like binge eating and your appearance. It helps you to challenge these beliefs which are unrealistic. Take for example, you may believe that you cannot control your eating or you are ugly and unattractive. This is not true. Therapy exposes you to real situations and helps you deal with them realistically. It changes what you belief and you become realistic.

Behavioral therapy deals with your behavior which is influenced by your thoughts and feelings. If you think you are ugly, you hide from people. Therapy helps you to correct your negative actions. CBT has gained popularity among therapists and patients because of its ability to treat mental disorders successfully. It is practiced by general practitioners, psychologists, psychiatrists, social workers, nurses who have the necessary training in CBT.

Support for binge eating disorder and body dysmorphic disorder

You can choose a support group to help you. There are many groups, which include formal and formal ones. You can have private or individualized psychological therapy which is a one-on-one therapy for individuals such as CBT. Therapy takes place between the therapist and patient. Group therapy is therapy given to a group facing the same challenges. It is led by a trained therapist or volunteer. Anything that affects the group members may be discussed whether it is about binge eating or healthy eating. Members discuss about their experiences while giving and receiving advice as they support one other. Self-help books are self-explanatory. You can read them alone or with a support group and share ideas. Online courses can be taken alone or as part of a support group. Supervised self-help programs are guided by a professional by having regular contacts usually on phone.

Family Therapy and/or Group Therapy

Family support is very important in making any type of treatment a success. It is important that your family members understand what body dysmorphic disorder is and learn to recognize its signs and symptoms, so they can help you overcome the problem. Those who live with their parents and siblings can work as a team. At times, working towards recovery together works better because you have people to encourage you and people you are accountable to. This makes you to put more efforts to get better. Your spouse and children can also help you cope as you strive towards recovery. We all crave to love and be loved. The first place you can easily find love is at home. Your family loves you just the way you are. In case your problems started because of the way you were treated, you don't have to hold onto this all your life, forgive and let go. This will start the healing process.

Conclusion

I am sure by now you have learnt a lot about body dysmorphic disorder and binge eating disorder. You can apply the steps we have recommended in this book to get better and overcome these problems regardless whether they started recently or they have been there for many years. There is hope for you and your loved ones who have these conditions. You should therefore be encouraged that you can overcome these problems and stop them from controlling your life.

You should know that you are not alone in your road to recovery. There are many people who are willing to help you. Look around you it may be your parents, spouse, siblings, close friends, doctors and therapists who are there to help you overcome your disorders. They may have noted that you have a problem but up to this time you may not have realized how important it is to get support.

If you have body dysmorphic disorder and/or binge eating disorder, you don't have to feel hopeless or worthlessness. There are many people who have applied what we have recommended in this book and they have achieved full recovery. That is why reading through the whole book and recommending it to other people who you care about will be of great benefit to you and to others. Don't hide your problems. Everyone you see has a problem although it may be different from yours. Take heart and strive towards recovery. You will recover and go on to have a happy and meaningful life.

I hope this book has helped you.